100 Questions & Answers About Lung Cancer

THIRD EDITION

Third edition

Joan H. Schiller, MD

Professor and Chief, Division of Hematology and Oncology
Deputy Director of Simmons Comprehensive Cancer Center
Andrea L. Simmons Distinguished Chair in Cancer Research
University of Texas Southwestern Medical Center
Dallas, Texas
and
President, National Lung Cancer Partnership
Madison, Wisconsin

Amy Cipau, MBA

President, North Carolina Lung Cancer Partnership
Raleigh, North Carolina
and
Vice President, National Lung Cancer Partnership
Madison, Wisconsin

JONES & BARTLETT
LEARNING

World Headquarters
Jones & Bartlett Learning
5 Wall Street
Burlington, MA 01803
978-443-5000
info@jblearning.com
www.jblearning.com

Jones & Bartlett Learning books and products are available through most bookstores and online booksell-ers. To contact Jones & Bartlett Learning directly, call 800-832-0034, fax 978-443-8000, or visit our website, www.jblearning.com.

Substantial discounts on bulk quantities of Jones & Bartlett Learning publications are available to corpora-tions, professional associations, and other qualified organizations. For details and specific discount informa-tion, contact the special sales department at Jones & Bartlett Learning via the above contact information or send an email to specialsales@jblearning.com.

100 Questions and Answers About Lung Cancer, Third Edition is an independent publication and has not been autho-rized, sponsored, or otherwise approved by the owners of the trademarks or service marks referenced in this product.

Some images in this book feature models. These models do not necessarily endorse, represent, or participate in the activities represented in the images.

The screenshots in this product are for educational and instructive purposes only. All trademarks displayed are the trademarks of the parties noted therein. Such use of trademarks is not an endorsement by said parties of Jones & Bartlett Learning, its products, or its services, nor should such use be deemed an endorsement by Jones & Bartlett Learning of said third party's products or services.

The authors, editor, and publisher have made every effort to provide accurate information. However, they are not responsible for errors, omissions, or for any outcomes related to the use of the contents of this book and take no responsibility for the use of the products and procedures described. Treatments and side effects described in this book may not be applicable to all people; likewise, some people may require a dose or experience a side effect that is not described herein. Drugs and medical devices are discussed that may have limited availability controlled by the Food and Drug Administration (FDA) for use only in a research study or clinical trial. Research, clinical practice, and government regulations often change the accepted standard in this field. When consideration is being given to use of any drug in the clinical setting, the health care provider or reader is responsible for deter-mining FDA status of the drug, reading the package insert, and reviewing prescribing information for the most up-to-date recommendations on dose, precautions, and contraindications, and determining the appropriate usage for the product. This is especially important in the case of drugs that are new or seldom used.

Production Credits
Executive Publisher: Christopher Davis
Editorial Assistant: Marisa LaFleur
Production Assistant: Alex Schab
Manufacturing and Inventory Control Supervisor:
   Amy Bacus
Marketing Associate: Jean O'Neil
Composition: Jason Miranda, Spoke & Wheel

Cover Design: Carolyn Downer
Cover Images: Top Left: © imagesource/123R;
   Top Right: © Jupiterimages/Comstock/
   Thinkstock; Bottom: © BananaStock/Thinkstock
Printing and Binding: Edwards Brothers Malloy
Cover Printing: Edwards Brothers Malloy

ISBN: 978-1-4496-8757-1

Library of Congress Cataloging-in-Publication Data
Schiller, J. H. (Joan H.), 1954–
  100 questions and answers about lung cancer / Joan H. Schiller, Amy Cipau. — Third edition.
     pages cm. — (100 questions and answers)
  ISBN 978-1-4496-8757-1 (alk. paper)
1. Lungs—Cancer—Popular works. I. Cipau, Amy. II. Title. III. Title: One hundred questions and answers about lung cancer.
  RC280.L8P365 2013
  616.99'424—dc23
                  2012037123
6048
Printed in the United States of America
16 15 14 13 12   10 9 8 7 6 5 4 3 2 1

*Dedicated to all lung cancer patients
and their caregivers.*

CONTENTS

Part 9: Living with Lung Cancer

Questions 85–92 provide practical advice on lifestyle choices or changes that you could encounter following a lung cancer diagnosis:

- How should I change my diet following a lung cancer diagnosis? Should I take dietary supplements? Can diet affect my survival from lung cancer?
- If I smoke, is there any reason to quit? How can I quit smoking while dealing with the stress of lung cancer?
- Should I be exercising?

Part 10: If Treatment Fails

Questions 93–96 address the difficult issues that arise if treatment options fail:

- How do I decide if it's time to stop treatment?
- What is hospice?
- What can I do to prepare for my death?

Part 11: Prevention, Screening, and Advocacy

Questions 97–100 discuss a variety of options for prevention, ways to screen for lung cancer, and advocacy:

- Can lung cancer be prevented? What is chemoprevention?
- Does lung cancer run in families? Is my family at increased risk for lung cancer because I have lung cancer?
- Why has there been so little progress in fighting lung cancer? What can I do to help?

Appendix: *Where Can I Find More Information?*

Glossary

Index

Getting a lung cancer diagnosis today is very different than it was a decade ago—today there is so much more hope! Over the last several years, new treatments for lung cancer have been developed and tested. New surgical techniques that cause less pain and shorter recoveries have become more widely available. New radiation-focusing devices ensure that only the tumor, and not the healthy tissue surrounding it, gets treated. Additional chemotherapy agents and targeted therapies—medicines designed to specifically attack cancer cells—have brought new treatment opportunities for the people diagnosed with this disease.

This book provides an overview of lung cancer for the person looking for a deeper understanding of the treatments for lung cancer, how to cope with the diagnosis, and the side effects associated with treatment. Receiving a lung cancer diagnosis can be scary and life changing, but a key part of living with lung cancer is to learn the facts and to stay positive and hopeful. *100 Questions & Answers About Lung Cancer, Third Edition* is designed to answer some of the most common questions patients and their loved ones have, while also providing sources for additional information.

The information found here will also help you understand how important it is to take an active role in making treatment-related decisions. A very significant decision for anyone entering lung cancer treatment is to consider whether participating in a clinical trial is right for them. Those who participated in clinical trials in the past have made possible the treatment advances of today. Further treatment advances and cures cannot happen unless patients get involved in clinical research.

If you are interested in taking part in a clinical trial and your doctor does not discuss this option with you, ask whether there might be an opportunity for you to participate.

Most importantly, perhaps, this book lets you know that you are not alone. There are more than 200,000 Americans diagnosed with lung cancer each year. There are peers for you to speak with and support groups to lean on. Organizations providing support resources can be found in the Appendix of this book.

Immense progress has been made in understanding lung cancer, but there is still a tremendous amount we do not know about the disease. Dr. Schiller and her colleagues founded the National Lung Cancer Partnership (*www.NationalLungCancerPartnership.org*) to increase the amount of funding available for lung cancer research and to raise awareness that lung cancer can happen to anyone—young or old, male or female, people with and without smoking histories. The Partnership is working to empower patients so they can make the best possible treatment choices, educate doctors to increase their ability to diagnose the disease earlier and provide the best available treatments, and raise awareness among the public to dispel the notion that this disease is self-inflicted and therefore unworthy of support. The Partnership also directly funds lung cancer research to bring new screening, diagnosis, treatment, and symptom management options to patients and trains advocates to raise the profile of lung cancer in their communities in an effort to increase the level of funding for this disease.

Other cancers have seen great strides in awareness and, consequently, research funding. For example, successes in breast cancer screening, treatment, and care came about because devoted, caring people joined together to raise awareness of the disease and funds for research. We need the same for lung cancer. We need people who have been affected by lung cancer to tell their stories, write to their congressional representatives, and work to raise awareness of and to support research funding for lung cancer. The National Lung Cancer Partnership's *Free to Breathe*® lung cancer awareness event series (*www.FreetoBreathe.org*)

is designed around this need; the number of events and participants are growing each year, bringing greater attention to this challenging disease to many local communities.

By reading this book, you'll have taken the first step toward understanding lung cancer. When you arm yourself with knowledge about the disease, you enable yourself to take charge of your care and your life.

Regina Vidaver, PhD
Executive Director
National Lung Cancer Partnership

The Basics

What is cancer?

What should I know about cancer cells?

How do normal lungs function?

More . . .

1. What is cancer?

Cancer cells differ from normal cells in a number of important ways. First, they are often unable to stop growing and divid-ing (unregu-lated growth). Second, cancer cells often stop doing their thing. In fact, they often stop doing anything useful at all.

Cancer is uncontrolled growth of **cells**—the billions upon billions upon billions of microscopic units that make up all the organs of our body. Cells are easily dis-tinguished from each other. Lung cells are very different in appearance from colon cells, for example, and do very different things. Colon cells are very different from blood cells, which are very different from muscle cells, and so forth. To understand what cancer is, you must first understand what makes a normal cell normal.

Normal cells do their own thing. For example, red blood cells carry oxygen throughout the body, stomach cells absorb nutrients, and **white blood cells** fight infections. Normal cells also stop growing and dividing when they get too old. In addition, normal cells often self destruct (undergo **apoptosis**) and die if they are injured.

Cancer cells differ from normal cells in a number of important ways. First, they are often unable to stop growing and dividing (unregulated growth). Second, cancer cells often stop doing their thing. In fact, they often stop doing anything useful at all. For example, cancerous white blood cells often stop fighting infection, stomach cancer cells stop absorbing nutrients, and lung cancer cells are unable to absorb oxygen. Another prop-erty of cancer cells is that they do not die like normal cells do when they grow old; they are literally immortal. In addition, cancer cells often spread to other organs, a process called **metastasis**. They can metastasize either by invading a nearby organ or by entering into the bloodstream or **lymphatic system** and traveling through the body to invade distant organs. Cancer cells can also make substances similar to hormones (called **growth**

factors) which can stimulate other cancer or normal cells to grow (see Question 2).

A **tumor** is a mass of tissue formed by a new growth of cells. If a tumor stops growing by itself, and does not invade other tissues, it is considered **benign**. Examples include lipomas, which are soft, spongy, fatty tumors that form just under the skin. Most tumors are **malignant**, which means they exhibit all the properties of cancer cells we've just mentioned.

Cancer can vary widely in terms of the malignant features we've just described—both between different types of cancers (e.g., leukemia vs. prostate cancer vs. breast cancer, etc.), and between people with the same type of cancer. For example, some types of cancers are very fast growing (e.g., acute leukemia) whereas others are usually much more slow growing (e.g., chronic leukemia). Some types tend to spread early on in their course (e.g., small cell lung cancer) whereas others tend to invade adjacent tissues (e.g., soft tissue sarcomas). Some manage to still retain some of the features of the tissues in which they arose (**well-differentiated** tumors) whereas others look so abnormal that the pathologist cannot tell where they came from by looking at them under a microscope (**poorly differentiated** tumors). Well-differentiated tumors tend to be slower growing and less aggressive, whereas poorly differentiated tumors often tend to grow and spread quickly. Thus, it is important that you realize that how someone else's breast cancer behaved, for example, is totally irrelevant to how your lung cancer is likely to behave—in terms of spread, growth rate, treatment, response to treatment, just about everything (see Question 12).

THE BASICS

Metastasis

The spread of cancer from the initial cancer site to other parts of the body.

Lymphatic system

A vascular system that contains lymph nodes through which white blood cells flow; cancer can also spread through the lymphatic system.

Growth factors

Substances that stimulate cells to grow; drugs that help the bone marrow recover from the effects of chemotherapy (see also colony-stimulating factors).

Tumor

A mass of tissue formed by a new growth of cells.

Benign

Not cancerous; not life threatening.

Malignant

Cancerous; cells that exhibit rapid, uncontrolled growth and can spread to other parts of the body.

Well-differentiated

Cancer cells which look relatively similar to the organ in which they started.

Poorly differentiated

Cancer cells that look wildly abnormal and nothing like the organ they started in.

Mutation

A damaged gene.

DNA (deoxyribonucleic acid)

Molecules that make up genes.

Chromosomes

Strands of DNA and proteins in the cell nucleus that are composed of a series of genes.

Nucleus

The center of the cell.

Gene

A section or sequence of DNA that regulates specific functions and is located in a specific place on a chromosome.

Carcinogens

Cancer-causing substances.

Just as different types of cancer vary in terms of how they behave (e.g., leukemia vs. prostate cancer vs. breast cancer), the same type of cancer will vary in its behavior from person to person. For example, in some patients a lung cancer might tend to spread, or metastasize early on, whereas in others it might not spread for a long time. Also, even the same type of cancers varies in terms of how they respond to treatment. Chemotherapy can be highly effective in shrinking the tumor in some patients with lung cancer, for example, whereas in others, chemotherapy might just stop the cancer from growing or not work at all (the cancer could be totally resistant to it). Why cancers differ depending on the tumor type, and why cancers behave differently from patient to patient, is an area of great interest with lots of research going on.

2. What should I know about cancer cells?

One generalization is that most cancer cells have **mutations** in their **DNA**. DNA is the brain of the cell. However, the DNA is not scattered diffusely throughout the cell; it is organized into 46 discrete units called **chromosomes**. The chromosomes are located in the center of the cell, the **nucleus**. Each cell in the human body contains 46 chromosomes. These chromosomes are made up of thousands of smaller units called **genes**; each of these genes regulates a particular function. For example, certain genes control the color of your hair. Others control how tall you grow; others control whether you produce insulin. If a gene is accidentally damaged, the change is called a mutation. It is not always clear what causes mutations. Some mutations are inherited, some could be due to diet, and others might be caused by exposure to environmental factors, such as radon or cancer-causing chemicals (**carcinogens**). For example, cigarette smoke contains hundreds of powerful carcinogens. Some mutations damage the gene or chromosome to the point where it causes the gene to stop working. This could result in the death of the cell, which is a relatively unusual cause of cancer. Cancer is usually due to the unregulated growth of cells, not their deaths.

Most mutations that cause cancer do so by causing the genes to work incorrectly. (Incidentally, many cancer cells from different patients have similar mutations.) Many of these mutations that cause cancer occur in genes that govern how cells grow or how cells die. After a normal gene is mutated, it is called either an **oncogene** or **tumor suppressor gene**. Oncogenes are genes that normally help cells grow. When they are mutated, they cannot shut off, and the cells cannot stop growing. (Something like the gas pedal of a car being pushed to the floor.) Tumor suppressor genes are genes that normally make injured or mutated cells stop growing. If they become mutated, they usually stop functioning, thus allowing the abnormal cells to continue to grow without stopping (as if the brakes of a car stopped working).

Oncogene

A gene that, when mutated, can allow a cell to grow uncontrollably.

Tumor suppressor gene

A gene that can normally block cancer from developing; when mutated, it cannot stop the growth of abnormal cells.

We also know that growth factors can be important in the development of cancer. Growth factors are substances made by cancer cells or (sometimes) normal cells. Estrogen, for example, is a growth factor made in the ovaries that is required for breast and ovarian cells to function normally. However, it can also cause some types of breast cancer cells to grow and divide. Some growth factors made by cancer cells tell other cells to grow and divide. An example of this is vascular epithelial growth factor (VEGF), a growth factor made by cancer cells that stimulates growth of new blood vessels. This is one way that tumors encourage blood vessels to grow into them, another common characteristic of cancer, because tumors often need blood vessels to support their growth. Except in certain circumstances, such as wound healing or pregnancy, new blood vessels rarely form in adults. Blood vessels are necessary for a tumor to grow because they deliver oxygen and nutrients to the tumor. They can also sometimes serve as a highway for tumor cells to travel as they spread throughout the body. Formation of new blood vessels is sometimes called **angiogenesis** (angio = blood; genesis = new; angiogenesis = formation). Another example of a growth factor is epidermal growth factor (EGF). (See Question 46.)

Angiogenesis

The formation of new blood vessels that allows tumors to grow.

3. Why do I need to know about genes? I'm not a doctor or a scientist!

True—but this is the age of molecular medicine. What that means is that, finally, all the research scientists have been doing all these years is starting to pay off. For decades scientists have been trying to figure out what makes a cancer cell differ from a normal cell, and they are finding out that the major difference is in the DNA of the cell. Most cancer cells have mutations in their DNA (Question 2), which makes an otherwise normal cell start to do some very abnormal things. Interestingly, there are some mutations found in many different types of cancer. There are other genes which, when mutated, cause a very specific type of cancer. (EGFR is an example of a mutated gene that only causes lung cancer.) More commonly, however, there are multiple genes found in a cancer that are mutated, and figuring out which genes are the important ones can be difficult. The study of looking at a lot of genes in many different types of cancer, or multiple genes in the tumors from many patients with the same cancer, is called **genomics**.

Genomics

The study of all mutations in a tumor to identify patterns that can be used to predict which tumors are more or less likely to respond to chemotherapy.

Because there are so many genes with so many mutations, in so many cancers, scientists often use statisticians to help them sort out all the data. The hope is that someday soon scientists will be able to identify which genes are critical ones for causing normal tissue to turn into lung cancer so that we can design drugs to target that particular set of abnormal genes.

4. How do normal lungs function?

Lungs are necessary for breathing—that is, bringing oxygen into the body and getting rid of carbon dioxide. Oxygen is necessary for cells to make energy. As this happens, the oxygen is used up and carbon dioxide is made. Carbon dioxide is a waste product, which needs to be removed from the body. This important oxygen-carbon dioxide exchange takes place in the lungs.

When we breathe in, or inhale, air travels through the main breathing tube called the **trachea**, which divides into two tubes (**main stem bronchi**) in the area near the heart. One tube goes to the right lung (right main stem bronchus) and the other to the left (left main stem bronchus). From there, the bronchi divide into smaller and smaller segments until they eventually become so tiny and thin that they are called alveoli. **Alveoli** are the millions of microscopic air sacs through which oxygen diffuses into red blood cells in the blood, where it is carried throughout the body. In exchange, carbon dioxide carried by the red blood cells from the body diffuses into the alveoli; it is then expelled out of the body through the airways when we exhale.

Notice that each lung is divided into sections called **lobes**. The right lung has three lobes, but the left lung

THE BASICS

Trachea
Breathing tube (airway) leading from the larynx to the lungs.

Main stem bronchi
The two main breathing tubes (right main stem bronchus and left main stem bronchus) that branch off the trachea.

Alveoli
Tiny air sacs that compose the lungs.

Lobes
Clear anatomical divisions or extensions that can be determined without the use of a microscope (at the gross anatomy level). The right lung contains three lobes and the left contains two.

has only two to make room for the heart. The heart assists in the vital process of breathing by pumping blood to and from the lungs (**Figure 1**).

Lymph node

Small collections of white blood cells scattered throughout the body.

Also notice that there are **lymph nodes** in the lung and in the space between the heart and the lung. These are important because lung cancers tend to spread via the lymphatic system. It is important that the surgeon biopsy these lymph nodes because if they do have cancer in them it would change the prognosis and treatment

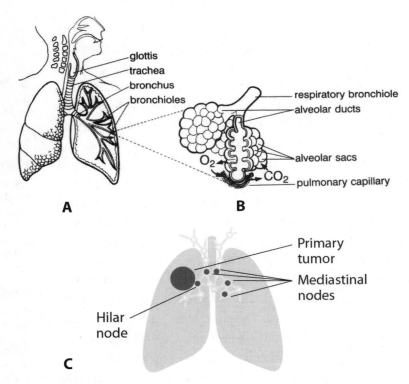

Figure 1 Internal structure of the lungs. **A.** Relationship of the lungs to the head and neck. **B.** External and internal appearance of a lung lobule, showing the alveolar sacs. **C.** Location of some representative hilar and mediastinal lymph nodes.

Parts A and B: Reprinted from Anderson PD and Spitzer VM. *Human Anatomy and Physiology Coloring Workbook and Study Guide*, Third Edition. Sudbury, MA: Jones and Bartlett Publishers, LLC, 2009.

Part C: Courtesy of the National Lung Cancer Partnership.

(see Question 11). The most common lymph nodes are nodes in the lung (lobar nodes) or right where the lung begins (**hilar lymph nodes**), often called N1 nodes, or in the space between the lung cancer the heart (**mediastinal lymph nodes, or N2 nodes**).

5. Are there different types of lung cancer?

There are four major types of lung cancer: **squamous cell carcinoma, adenocarcinoma, large cell carcinoma**, and **small cell carcinoma**. The primary difference between squamous cell, adenocarcinoma, and large cell carcinoma is how they look under the microscope. These three are sometimes collectively called **non-small cell lung cancer** (**NSCLC**) to distinguish them from **small cell lung cancer** (**SCLC**), or small cell carcinoma. In the United States, adenocarcinoma is the most common type of lung cancer, representing about 40% of all lung cancers. Sometimes, it is difficult to tell what type of NSCLC it is, in which case it might be called poorly differentiated or NSCLC—not otherwise specified (NSCLC-NOS).

Small cell lung cancer represents roughly 15%–20% of all lung cancers. It differs from the three types of non-small cell lung cancer in several important ways. It tends to be more rapidly growing, causes symptoms quicker, and spreads more rapidly. SCLC also tends to be more sensitive to **chemotherapy** and **radiation therapy** than NSCLC. For these reasons, patients with SCLC rarely undergo surgery. Instead, the standard treatment is chemotherapy, sometimes with radiation therapy (see Question 55).

THE BASICS

Hilar lymph nodes
Lymph nodes located in the region where the bronchus meets the lung.

Mediastinal lymph nodes
Lymph nodes located in the mediastinum, the area between the lungs.

N2 nodes
Mediastinal nodes (e.g., nodes between the lungs and the heart).

There are four major types of lung cancer: squamous cell carcinoma, adenocarcinoma, large cell carcinoma, and small cell carcinoma.

Squamous cell carcinoma
A type of non-small cell lung cancer.

Adenocarcinoma
A type of non-small cell lung cancer; a malignant tumor that arises from glandular tissue.

Large cell carcinoma

A type of non-small cell lung cancer.

Small cell carcinoma

A type of lung cancer that differs in appearance and behavior from non-small cell lung cancers (adenocarcinoma, squamous cell carcinoma, large cell carcinoma).

Non-small cell lung cancer (NSCLC)

A type of lung cancer that includes adenocarcinoma, squamous cell carcinoma, and large cell carcinoma.

Small cell lung cancer (SCLC)

Refers to small cell carcinoma, as opposed to non-small cell lung cancers (adenocarcinoma, squamous cell carcinoma, large cell carcinoma).

Chemotherapy

The use of medicine to treat cancer; a whole-body or systemic treatment.

Radiation therapy

Treatment that uses high-dose X-rays or other high-energy rays to kill cancer cells.

Until very recently, squamous cell carcinoma, adenocarcinoma, and large cell carcinoma were all treated the same way. However, more recent data suggests that some treatments might be more effective or safer in one subtype than another, such as bevacizumab or pemetrexed (see Question 43).

One sub-type of adenocarcinoma also bears mentioning: **Adenocarcinoma-in-situ** (**AIS**, formerly known as **bronchioloalveolar carcinoma**, or **BAC**). AIS is a rare form of lung cancer, representing only about 5% of all lung cancers. For unknown reasons, the number of patients developing AIS is rising. AIS is unique in that it tends to spread diffusely throughout the alveoli (see Question 4), unlike the more typical lung cancer cells which tend to stick together and form solid, discrete masses. The cause of AIS is less clear than for other forms of lung cancer. AIS tends to occur in younger, nonsmoking women. Of all the types of lung cancer, it is the one that is most often found in patients who have never smoked, although it is also found in smokers.

6. What causes lung cancer?

Eighty-five to 90% of lung cancers are caused by carcinogens in tobacco that cause damage (mutations) to the DNA in lung cells. People are usually exposed to these carcinogens by directly inhaling them while smoking; however, people can sometimes develop lung cancer because they have inhaled large quantities of smoke from other smokers (**passive smoking**). Rarely, radon (a gas found underground) can also cause lung cancer. Exposure to asbestos, air pollution, and certain other environmental carcinogens can also cause lung cancer. When this occurs, it is usually a result of long-term, occupational exposure. (See Questions 97–99 for information on lung cancer risk, screening, and prevention.) However, sometimes people who have never smoked and do not have a history of exposure to any of these environmental carcinogens also get lung cancer. More research is needed to determine why these individuals get lung cancer.

7. Who gets lung cancer? Is it contagious? Can my children get it from me?

Lung cancer is second only to prostate cancer in men and breast cancer in women in **incidence** (incidence is the number of new patients who develop a cancer in 1 year per 100,000 people). Unfortunately, lung cancer is the leading cause of cancer death among both men and women and is responsible for more cancer-related deaths than breast cancer, colon cancer, and prostate cancer combined.

Lung cancer is most commonly found in current or former smokers, usually in their late 60s. The incidence of lung cancer has been on the rise since smoking became popular in the 1920s and 1930s, but it began to rise rapidly around 1960 when the effects of the cigarette boom during the World War II years became evident. The death rate for lung cancer in men peaked in the late 1980s; however, it continued to rise in women until roughly the year 2000, when it started to level off. Many people do not realize that lung cancer is the leading cancer killer of both men and women. Of note, although stopping smoking significantly decreases the risk of lung cancer, the risk never goes down to zero. Approximately 50% of all lung cancers occur in former smokers. This does not mean that it does not matter

Adenocarcinoma-in-situ (AIS)

Formerly called bronchoalveolar carcinoma, a subtype of adenocarcinoma sometimes found in non-smokers.

Bronchioloalveolar carcinoma (now called Adenocarcinoma-in-situ (AIS)

A type of adenocarcinoma.

Passive smoking

Inhaling cigarette smoke of others.

Incidence

The number of new cases of a cancer (or any disease or event) in a defined population during a set period of time.

if one quits smoking or not. Even if the risk of lung cancer never goes down to zero, it still drops precipitously. In addition, there are multiple other health benefits to quitting smoking, such as a reduction in heart disease, hypertension, etc.

For reasons we do not understand, occasionally people who have never smoked get lung cancer. An estimated 15% of lung cancer patients in the United States have never smoked. In certain areas of the world, the percentage is much higher. For example, in Asia the majority of women who get lung cancer have never smoked.

Please note that lung cancer is **NOT** contagious. No one can catch it from you. It is also not inheritable; lung cancer cannot be passed down from one generation to another.

Diagnosis and Staging

What are the most common symptoms of lung cancer?

How is lung cancer diagnosed?

What is staging, and why is it important?

More . . .

8. What are the most common symptoms of lung cancer?

The symptoms of lung cancer depend upon its location. If a cancer occurs near the center of the chest, for example, it often presses on a major airway or blood vessel. In these cases, common symptoms include cough (including blood-tinged **sputum**) and shortness of breath. If the tumor blocks or obstructs a major airway, bacteria and secretions can back up behind the obstruction, resulting in a post-obstructive **pneumonia**.

Other structures near the center of the chest are sometimes affected by lung cancer. Rarely, the recurrent laryngeal nerve might be involved. The recurrent laryngeal nerve is a nerve that goes from the brain to the vocal cords. Because of the way humans develop as fetuses this nerve does not make a direct path from the brain to the vocal cord, as one might expect. Instead, it travels down to the chest and then back up again, swinging by the major vessels leading in and out of the heart. If the tumor happens to press upon this nerve, hoarseness can result. Similarly, if the tumor happens to press on the **esophagus**, the feeding tube that leads from the mouth to the stomach, patients can experience problems with swallowing. If the tumor presses on one of the great vessels leading into the heart, such as the superior vena cava, the blood sometimes cannot flow easily into the heart. Instead, it backs up into the neck, shoulders, and arms (**superior vena cava syndrome [SVC]**). In this case, patients can experience swelling of these areas.

If the tumor arises farther out in the lung near the chest wall, patients can experience pain. Indeed, this is often

Sputum
Mucus and other secretions produced by the lungs.

Pneumonia
An infection of the lung.

Esophagus
The tube through which food travels from the mouth to the stomach.

Superior vena cava syndrome (SVCS)
A collection of symptoms that could include swelling in the neck, shoulders, and arms caused by a lung tumor pressing on the SVC, one of the large vessels leading into the heart.

the only time patients experience pain from lung cancer because this is really the only area of the lung that has nerve endings. The middle of the lung and the area near the heart do not have many nerve endings, so tumors that arise in these areas rarely cause pain. This is one of the reasons why lung cancer can grow unnoticed for a long period of time. It is painless unless the chest wall is involved.

Tumors arising near the chest wall can also cause a **pleural effusion** (see Question 83). A pleural effusion is an accumulation of fluid between the outside of the lung and the inside of the chest wall. This fluid can cause pain, cough, and shortness of breath.

If the tumor occurs near the top of the lung, (**Pancoast tumor** or **superior sulcus tumor**) it could grow into some of the nerves leaving the spinal cord and travel down through the armpit and into the arm. In this case, it can cause shoulder pain or weakness, or an unusual group of symptoms consisting of a droopy eyelid, dry eyes, and lack of sweating on the face.

If the tumor metastasizes, its symptoms will be related to the area of the body to which it has spread. For example, if the cancer spreads to the bone, it could cause pain in the back, hip, leg, or arm. If it spreads to the brain, it can cause headaches, nausea, or signs and symptoms similar to a stroke. These symptoms are not unique to metastatic lung cancer—any cancer that spreads to these organs will cause similar symptoms. The most frequent symptoms of cancer, however, are fatigue, weakness, loss of appetite, and weight loss. These symptoms often indicate that the cancer is advanced.

Pleural effusion

Accumulation of fluid between the outside of the lung and the inside of the chest wall.

Superior sulcus tumor

See pancoast tumor.

Pancoast tumor (superior sulcus tumor)

A tumor occurring near the top of the lungs that may cause shoulder pain or weakness or a group of symptoms including a droopy eyelid, dry eyes, and lack of sweating on the face.

The most frequent symptoms of cancer, however, are fatigue, weakness, loss of appetite, and weight loss. These symptoms often indicate that the cancer is advanced.

DIAGNOSIS AND STAGING

9. Are there other symptoms associated with lung cancer?

Paraneoplastic symptoms

Symptoms that result from substances released by cancer cells and that occur at a site not directly involved with the tumor.

Electrolytes

Acids, bases, and salts essential for maintaining life; electrolyte abnormalities are imbalances of salts or chemicals in the blood.

Neuropathy

See peripheral neuropathy.

Clubbing

A condition that causes the nails on the fingers to bulge out; clubbing occurs with many different types of lung problems.

X-ray

High-energy radiation used to image the body.

Sometimes tumors can cause **paraneoplastic symptoms**. Paraneoplastic symptoms occur at a site not directly involved with the tumor. Presumably, the tumor must be making some type of hormone to affect these distant sites. Common paraneoplastic syndromes include **electrolyte** abnormalities (such as calcium and sodium imbalances), **neuropathy** (numbness and tingling of the hands and feet), and **clubbing** of the fingers. Clubbing can occur with many different types of lung problems (not only lung cancer). It is a word for the situation when the nails on the fingers bulge out somewhat. The cause of this effect is not known.

Patients with cancer are more susceptible to blood clots in the legs (deep venous thromboses, or DVTs). This is a paraneoplastic syndrome that occurs when tumors generate substances that make the blood more prone to clotting.

10. How is lung cancer diagnosed?

The diagnosis of lung cancer frequently is made when a patient goes to his or her primary care physician complaining of cough, shortness of breath, and low-grade fevers. Because these symptoms are so common, the patient is often treated for a bronchitis or respiratory infection with antibiotics without taking a chest **X-ray**. If the symptoms do not go away, however, a chest X-ray is eventually obtained, revealing some type of mass in the chest. The X-ray is frequently followed by a chest CT scan to provide a better picture of the lungs and chest. This, in turn, often results in a **biopsy** (sampling of tissue), which is required for diagnosis of any type of cancer. (CT scan and biopsy are discussed further in Question 11.)

Biopsy

Removal of tissue or fluid sample for microscopic examination.

11. Which tests are performed to diagnose lung cancer?

A computed tomography or CT scan (sometimes called a CAT scan) is the most helpful test for visualizing an abnormality in the lung. CT scans are a series of X-rays in which the body is sliced up like a pack of Lifesavers. Each one of the slices is then called up on a computer screen to give a cross-sectional image of the chest. A CT scan offers considerably more detail than a regular chest X-ray. To help the radiologist distinguish between blood vessels and tumors on CT scans, a dye called CT or IV contrast is sometimes injected into the vein to make the blood vessels more pronounced.

Once a suspicious abnormality is found on a CT scan, the patient needs a biopsy to obtain a diagnosis. There are several ways of doing this:

- **Bronchoscopy.** A bronchoscopy is a procedure in which a lung doctor (**pulmonologist**) inserts a flexible tube called a **bronchoscope** through the nose down into the lungs. The bronchoscope, which has fiber optic lighting inside, has several purposes. It can serve as a periscope, allowing the pulmonologist to see into the airways. Additionally, needles can be inserted through the bronchoscope to obtain biopsies. The procedure is usually done on an outpatient basis, under sedation.

Bronchoscopy

A procedure that involves inserting a flexible tube (bronchoscope) through the nose down into the lungs. Needles can be inserted through the bronchoscope to obtain biopsy samples.

Pulmonologist

A physician who specializes in the diagnosis and treatment of lung diseases.

Bronchoscope

See Bronchoscopy.

Although bronchoscopy is a commonly used diagnostic test, it does have several disadvantages. First, the pulmonologist usually cannot get the tube into the distant areas of the lung—the airways near the chest wall are too small for the bronchoscope to get through. Therefore, the use of this test is limited to the larger bronchi, or airways. Second, if the cancer itself is not actually growing in the airway, it can be difficult for the pulmonologist to get a biopsy because he or she cannot actually see the tumor.

Alternatives

- **Transthoracic (percutaneous) biopsy.** Specialized doctors, called **interventional radiologist**s, can sometimes insert a needle from the outside in— through the skin and chest wall into the tumor—in order to obtain tissue for a biopsy. This procedure usually does not require a hospital stay (it is an outpatient procedure) and is often done under a local anesthetic.

- **Surgery.** Sometimes the abnormality seen on chest X-ray or CT scan cannot be easily biopsied by either a bronchoscopy or a transthoracic biopsy. In this case, patients might have to undergo a relatively minor surgical procedure under general anesthetic (and thus might require an overnight stay in the hospital). The surgeon can do several different procedures to make the diagnosis. These include:

  – **Mediastinoscopy.** This procedure involves making a small incision above the collarbone or between the spaces of the first and second or second and third ribs. The surgeon then inserts a special tube through this incision into the **mediastinum**. Again, this tube has two functions: it allows the surgeon to see the lymph

Transthoracic (percutaneous) biopsy

A biopsy in which a needle is inserted from the outside into the tumor.

Interventional radiologist

A radiologist who uses X-rays and other imaging techniques to perform minimally invasive medical procedures.

Surgery

Removal of tissue by means of an operation (surgical procedure).

Mediastinoscopy

A surgical procedure by which lymph nodes can be removed for microscopic examination.

Mediastinum

Area between the lungs.

nodes near the heart, and it also allows the surgeon to biopsy them. A mediastinoscopy is sometimes done not only to make the diagnosis of cancer but also to help stage the patient (see Question 15).

- **Video-assisted thoracoscopic surgery (VATS).** This procedure involves making a small incision someplace on the outside of the chest and inserting a fiber optic tube into the space between the chest wall and the lung. This allows a surgeon to see the outside of the lung and to biopsy any suspicious areas.

- **Robotic surgery.** No, this does not mean the surgery is carried out by a robot! This is similar to a VATS procedure except the fiber optic instruments are smaller. For the surgeon to be able to manipulate them, he or she sits at a console and uses devices that look something like a joystick on a video game.

12. What results will my doctor get from the biopsy?

It typically takes 2 to 3 days before the biopsy results become available. We strongly suggest that you schedule an appointment with your doctor to receive the results and discuss your **prognosis** and treatment options. There is nothing worse than getting bad news over the phone, especially when the doctor might not have much time to talk to you.

Video-assisted thoracoscopic surgery (VATS)

A type of minimally invasive chest surgery.

Robotic surgery

A type of minimally invasive surgery, in which the surgeon manipulates the instruments from a console that does not have to be next to the patient's bed.

It typically takes 2 to 3 days before the biopsy results become available.

Prognosis

Predicted outcome; likelihood of survival.

Pathologist

A physician trained to examine and evaluate cells and tissue.

A specialized doctor called a **pathologist** looks at the biopsy samples under the microscope. He or she tries to answer the following critical questions:

- First, is it cancer? The pathologist determines this by judging how normal the cells look. Part of the definition of cancer is that cancer cells look very abnormal and no longer look or function like the type of cells they are supposed to be. However, the question as to whether something is cancerous is not always as black or white as one might suppose. Typically, normal cells from different parts of our body look very different microscopically and are easy to tell apart—blood cells look very different from muscle cells, for example. In some tumors, however, the cells are so wildly abnormal looking that one cannot tell where they originated from or from what part of the body they were taken. In this case, cells are called poorly differentiated. In other cases the cells might look abnormal (but you can still tell where they came from) and in others only somewhat abnormal (e.g., they only look a little different from normal cells). Pathologists use the term **differentiation** to describe the degree of abnormality of the appearance of the cells. A well-differentiated adenocarcinoma, for example, looks somewhat like normal lung cells. Generally speaking, the more differentiated a cancer looks, the less aggressive it is likely to be.

Differentiation

A term used to describe the degree to which tumor tissue resembles normal tissue.

- If it is cancer, what kind is it? As discussed in Question 5, there are four major types of lung cancer (adenocarcinoma, squamous cell carcinoma, large cell carcinoma, or small cell carcinoma). While typing is based on the cancer's appearance microscopically, the most important distinction is whether or not it is small cell lung cancer.

Pathologists classify tumors into different **histological** types based upon the characteristics or patterns some tumors make when looked at under the microscope. For example, adenocarcinomas often look like glands; large cell carcinomas contain—you guessed it—large cancer cells; and small cell cancers contain small cancer cells. As it turns out, many cancers that start in different parts of the body can also look glandular. For example, breast cancer, colon cancer, and prostate cancers are also adenocarcinomas. Sometimes, they are hard to tell apart, so the pathologist will stain the tumor with special stains. For example, breast cancer cells tend to stain positive for the estrogen receptor (ER), whereas most lung adenocarcinomas stain positive for Thyroid Transcription Factor 1 (**TTF1**). If a poorly differentiated adenocarcinoma stains negative for ER but positive for TTF1, the pathologist is more likely to conclude that the tumor rose in the lungs and not in the breast.

- If it is cancer, where did it come from? If a tumor starts in the lung, it is called lung cancer. However, other cancers commonly spread to the lungs. If a tumor starts elsewhere in the body, say, the breast, and spreads to the lung, it is still called breast cancer. If a lung cancer spreads to the liver, for example, it is still called lung cancer. This is because in general, cancers typically behave like the cancer where it came from—breast cancer that has spread or metastasized to the lung still tends to respond to breast cancer chemotherapy better than lung cancer chemotherapy and tends to grow and behave similarly to breast cancer elsewhere in the body.

Histological

Tissue type; assessment of cellular features by microscopic evaluation.

TTF1

A protein lung adenocarcinoma cells have on the outside of their membrane. Since it is primarily found on adenocarcinoma cells of the lung, and not other types of cancer, it is frequently used to tell if a cancer in the lung started in the lung (e.g., lung cancer) or whether it spread to the lung from some other organ (e.g., metastatsized to the lung).

DIAGNOSIS AND STAGING

13. Is it important to know what type of lung cancer I have?

In the past, we have generally treated all non-small cell carcinomas the same. More recently, however, there is data indicating that patients with squamous cell carcinoma might not respond as well to a type of chemotherapy called pemetrexed (Alimta). In addition, patients with squamous cell carcinoma are more likely to have side effects from bevacizumab (Avastin), so bevacizumab is rarely given to these patients. Also, adenocarcinomas tend to have different mutations than squamous or small cell lung cancer.

14. What are lymph nodes?

Lymph nodes are small collections of white blood cells scattered throughout the body. White blood cells not only flow through the bloodstream, they also flow through a second type of vascular system in our bodies called the lymphatic system. Unlike the other organs in our body, of which everyone has the same number (e.g., we all have two lungs, one liver, one heart), there are hundreds of different lymph nodes scattered throughout the body, and everyone has a slightly different number of them.

Lymph nodes are important because sometimes cancer can spread through the lymphatic system. If the lymph nodes that your surgeon removes contain cancer, this implies that since your lung cancer spread to the lymph nodes, it might also have passed through the lymph nodes and spread elsewhere in your body.

15. What is staging, and why is it important?

Staging a tumor involves determining where the tumor is, its size, and how far a cancer has spread. This is useful for several reasons:

- Staging allows physicians to have a common language in describing a patient's tumor. Thus, when a surgeon tells an oncologist that a patient has Stage IIIA lung cancer, the oncologist immediately has some idea as to the extent of the patient's disease.

- It is an important prognostic indicator. Patients with Stage I disease, for example, typically do much better than do patients with Stage IV disease.

- It is very useful for determining therapy. The type of treatment that is recommended—surgery, radiotherapy, chemotherapy, or any combination of these—will depend upon the extent of the disease and how far it has spread.

Staging

Determining the size of a cancer and how far it has spread.

16. What are the staging guidelines for NSCLC?

The staging of cancer is classically dependent upon three criteria: the size and location of the tumor (T or tumor status); whether any lymph nodes are involved (N or nodal status); and whether the cancer has spread further than the lymph nodes (M or metastatic status). These three criteria (T, N, and M) are further subdivided. For example, if no lymph nodes contain the tumor, this is called N0; if the local (hilar) lymph nodes contain the tumor, this is called N1; and if the lymph nodes between the lung and the heart (mediastinal lymph nodes) contain tumor, this is typically called N2. N3 disease

DIAGNOSIS AND STAGING

involves the lymph nodes in the other side of the chest or in the area above the collar bone.

Oncologists use a complicated system, based upon the TNM staging, to determine the overall stage. A simplified summary is provided in **Table 1**.

17. What are the staging guidelines for small cell lung cancer (SCLC)?

Because SCLC tends to metastasize early, oncologists typically do not go into the formal TNM staging classification noted above. Instead, they typically divide SCLC into limited stage or extensive stage disease, in which limited stage is defined as cancer confined to one

Table 1 Lung cancer staging based upon the TNM staging criteria

Stage I	Tumors that are small and do not have any lymph node involvement
Stage II	Larger tumors, or tumors that have spread to the local (hilar) lymph nodes, OR tumors abutting the chest wall without lymph node involvement
Stage III	Tumors that are "locally advanced" but do not appear to have metastasized to distant organs
Stage IIIA	Tumors that are large and bulky but are still surgically resectable (i.e., the surgeon is technically able to take the tumor out), OR tumors that have spread to the mediastinal lymph nodes
Stage IIIB	Tumors that have not yet metastasized, but that are too large to resect or that are located such that the surgeon would be unable to resect them safely. Typical examples are tumors that have invaded the heart, one of the large blood vessels leading into or out of the heart, or one of the major airways. Also, lymph node (see Question 14) involvement on the opposite side of the chest (N3) is classified as having Stage IIIB disease.
Stage IV	Tumors that have spread to other organs (metastasized), or have resulted in pleural effusions (see Question 83).

side of the chest, and extensive stage is defined as cancer that has spread outside the side of the chest from which it arose.

The most common metastatic sites for both non-small cell and small cell lung cancer are in the lungs, the liver, the adrenal glands, the bones, and the brain.

18. Which tests and procedures are used to detect whether my lung cancer has spread beyond my chest?

Your oncologist might order a series of tests to determine whether the cancer has spread to one of the sites mentioned above. These might include a **bone scan** (an imaging test in which a radionuclear substance is injected into the veins and taken up by cancer cells, if any, in the bones), a head or abdominal **CT scan**, or a **PET scan**. PET (positron emission tomography) is a nuclear medicine scan that measures metabolism or how quickly cells break down nutrients for energy. Because cancer cells grow faster than normal cells, they presumably need more energy than normal cells. Since cancer cells get their energy from sugar, or glucose, they are more likely to use more glucose than normal cells, a difference that can be picked up on a PET scan. PET scans are most often used at the time of diagnosis to help stage a patient. In particular, it is often used to help the surgeon to decide which lymph nodes might have cancer and therefore should be biopsied.

PET scans are not perfect, however. White blood cells also use a lot of glucose. Thus, any infection or irritation (inflammation) could also be positive on PET scan (false positive). In addition, broncheoalveolar cancers are

Bone scan

An imaging test in which a radionuclear substance is injected into the veins and taken up by the bones in areas of potential metastatic disease.

CT scan (computed tomography)

Computerized series of X-rays that create a detailed cross-sectional image of the body.

PET scan (positron emission tomography)

A nuclear medicine imaging test that measures metabolism; often used to differentiate between healthy and abnormal (e.g., cancerous) tissue.

sometimes so slow growing that they do not use a lot of glucose and thus can be falsely negative on PET scan. Finally, our brains use so much glucose that it is difficult to see a cancer or tumor in the brain on PET scan.

I've Just Been Diagnosed with Lung Cancer— Now What?

Who treats lung cancer?
What is multidisciplinary care?

Should I get a second opinion?

How can I relate best to my doctor? What can I do to make my medical visits as productive as possible?

More . . .

19. Who treats lung cancer? What is multidisciplinary care?

Multidisciplinary clinic

a multidisciplinary clinic is one in which doctors of different specialities—e.g. medical oncology, radiation oncology and surgeons—all see the patient within the same clinic.

Medical oncologist

A physician who performs comprehensive management of cancer patients throughout all phases of care; specializes in treating cancer with medicine.

Systemic

Affecting the entire body.

Lung cancer is a complex disease, and its treatment frequently involves some combination of surgery, chemotherapy, and radiation (see Questions 35, 40, and 47). You likely will see more than one specialist for your lung cancer care, including medical oncologists, thoracic surgeons, radiation oncologists, and pulmonologists. Ideally, these lung cancer doctors work together in a **multidisciplinary clinic** or other setting where they can easily consult together, with each other, about your treatment options. This multidisciplinary approach not only offers you high-quality care but also has practical advantages that might include fewer trips to the doctor, less time from diagnosis to start of treatment, and more efficient coordination of the logistics involving treatment. Multidisciplinary care is commonly offered in cancer centers and in larger treatment centers such as university hospitals, but it is beginning to be implemented in some community hospitals as well.

Each lung cancer specialist you see is a member of your treatment team, but one doctor (usually the medical oncologist) will have primary responsibility for managing and directing your care.

There are also a number of other doctors, along with support staff, who will be involved in your care. It is helpful to understand what each of these healthcare professionals does and what role he or she plays in your care.

- **Medical oncologist**: a physician who performs comprehensive management of cancer patients throughout all phases of care. Medical oncologists specialize in treating cancer with medicine, using **systemic** treatments such as chemotherapy.

- **Thoracic surgeon**: a surgeon who specializes in performing lung surgery. A thoracic surgeon might have performed the tumor biopsy that resulted in your lung cancer diagnosis. Some thoracic surgeons have received additional training in lung cancer surgery and are considered surgical oncologists.

- **Radiation oncologist**: a physician who specializes in treating cancer with radiation.

- **Pulmonologist**: a physician who specializes in the diagnosis and treatment of lung diseases. A pulmonologist might have diagnosed your lung cancer. You could also see a pulmonologist if you have ongoing respiratory issues related to your lung cancer or underlying conditions such as bronchitis, emphysema, or **chronic obstructive pulmonary disease (COPD)**.

Other specialists or support staff:

- **Pathologist**: a physician trained to examine and evaluate cells and tissue under the microscope. The pathologist evaluates your biopsy tissue and furnishes a biopsy report to your oncologist or surgeon.

- **Oncology nurse**: a specialized nurse trained to provide care to cancer patients, including administering chemotherapy and monitoring side effects.

- **Psychiatrist**: a physician who specializes in treating people for depression, anxiety, and other psychological illness. Psychiatrists provide psychotherapy and can also prescribe medication.

- **Psychologist**: a person trained in psychology who can provide psychotherapy or counseling to help patients and their families better cope with their disease.

- **Patient navigator**: a nurse, nurse practitioner, social worker or other healthcare personnel whose job is to

---

Thoracic surgeon

A surgeon who specializes in performing chest surgery.

Radiation oncologist

A physician who specializes in treating cancer with radiation.

Chronic obstructive pulmonary disease (COPD)

Chronic bronchitis or emphysema.

COPD

Chronic obstructive pulmonary disease. Emphysema and bronchitis are the two most common forms of COPD.

Oncology nurse

A specialized nurse trained to provide care to cancer patients.

Psychiatrist

A physician who specializes in treating people for depression, anxiety, and other psychological illness. Psychiatrists provide psychotherapy and can also prescribe medication.

Psychologist

A person trained in psychology who can provide psychotherapy or counseling to help patients and their families better cope with their disease.

Patient navigator

A nurse, nurse practitioner, social worker, or other healthcare personnel whose job is to coordinate your care (e.g., make sure all your questions are answered, your tests are scheduled, your treatments are on time, etc.).

Oncology social worker

A social worker trained to provide counseling and practical assistance to cancer patients.

Rehabilitation specialist

A person trained to help patients recover from physical changes brought about by cancer or cancer treatment.

coordinate your care (make sure all your questions are answered, your tests are scheduled, your treatments are on time, etc.) If your hospital or doctor's office is lucky enough to have a patient navigator, get this person's number! He or she will probably be your primary point person.

- **Oncology social worker**: a social worker trained to provide counseling and practical assistance to cancer patients. Social workers can help you locate services such as transportation, support groups, and home care. They can also provide assistance with insurance and financial issues.

- **Rehabilitation specialist**: a person trained to help patients recover from physical changes brought about by cancer or cancer treatment. Respiratory therapists help lung cancer patients to maximize their breathing capacity and learn to cope with breathlessness. Physical therapists can help patients recover range of motion and strength following lung cancer surgery.

- **Nutritionist** or **dietician**: a person trained to provide nutritional or dietary counseling. Lung cancer patients could experience weight loss as a result of their cancer or its treatment (see Question 85). Treatment side effects, such as nausea from chemotherapy or heartburn from radiation, can negatively affect appetite. Nutritional or dietary counseling services can help patients to increase appetite and gain weight.

- **Palliative care specialist**: a physician trained in managing cancer pain and other symptoms of cancer.

20. How do I find the best doctors to treat my lung cancer? Does the hospital make any difference in my care?

One of your primary responsibilities as a lung cancer patient is to be sure that you are getting the best care possible, starting with your choice of doctors. Although it is often difficult for patients to assess the quality of doctors and treatment centers, there are resources you can turn to, and questions you can ask, to help you decide on the right doctor for you.

The first step in finding a doctor or treatment center is to get a recommendation from a reliable source. Your primary care physician, or another doctor, can refer you to the best lung cancer specialists in your area. Other lung cancer patients are also good sources. If you cannot get a recommendation for a specific lung cancer specialist, you can contact the nearest cancer center or university hospital and ask for the names of their oncologists who specialize in lung cancer. The leading cancer centers are identified by the National Cancer Institute as NCI-designated cancer centers. The American College of Surgeons' Commission on Cancer also identifies hospitals with strong cancer programs. (For further information on these resources, and on others that will help you to locate doctors and cancer treatment centers, see the Appendix.)

After you have the name of a doctor, you need to evaluate whether this person is a quality physician. Equally important, you need to decide whether you are comfortable with this person and whether the two of you will be able to communicate well with each other as you face the difficult decisions that lie ahead.

Palliative care specialist

A physician trained in management of pain or other symptoms of cancer.

Nutritionist or dietician

A person trained to provide nutritional or dietary counseling.

One of your primary responsibilities as a lung cancer patient is to be sure that you are getting the best care possible, starting with your choice of doctors.

Some things to consider:

- *Experience or expertise in lung cancer.* It is extremely important to find out whether a physician has extensive experience with lung cancer patients. Oncologists treat patients with all types of cancers, but ideally you want to find an oncologist who specializes in lung cancer. This type of medical oncologist is referred to as a thoracic (or lung) oncologist and can be found at major cancer centers. Similarly, if you are seeking a surgeon you want to find a thoracic surgeon who specializes in lung cancer surgery and not a cardiac surgeon who specializes in heart surgery or a general surgeon who performs all types of surgeries. Studies have shown that the complication rate is lower for lung cancer surgery when the surgery is performed by a thoracic surgeon. You should ask any prospective oncologist or surgeon what percentage of his or her practice is lung cancer patients.

- *Hospital affiliation.* It is important to consider your doctor's hospital affiliation. Cancer centers and university hospitals conduct research and provide access to the newest treatments and to **clinical trials** (see Question 59). Patients are more likely to receive multidisciplinary care in these institutions and benefit from the collective expertise of multiple specialists. Patients who undergo surgery for lung cancer at hospitals that perform a large volume of lung surgery are likely to survive longer and have fewer complications than patients who have similar surgery at hospitals with a low volume of lung cancer procedures.

You should be aware that cancer centers and university hospitals tend to be larger than community hospitals and often have fellows (doctors who

Clinical trials

Research studies involving people.

are learning to be oncologists), residents (doctors in training), or medical students who see patients with the medical oncologist; however, even in these teaching hospitals your care will be directed by the medical oncologist who should be seeing you at every visit with the fellow or resident. This might seem confusing, especially at the beginning, but most people get used to these differences. Hospital affiliation should be a major factor in deciding who your physician will be.

- *Credentials.* Basic professional information for licensed U.S. physicians is available through the American Medical Association's Physician Select website, *www.ama-assn.org.* Each listing offers information on the physician's medical school, residency and fellowship training, board certification, and office location. Board certification ensures expertise in a specified area, such as medical oncology, radiation oncology, or thoracic surgery. Residency or fellowship training at a major cancer center can be a plus.

Other factors to consider:

- *Is the doctor covered by your insurance plan?* Financial constraints are a reality, and insurance is a limiting factor when selecting a doctor. There could be overriding reasons for consulting a specialist (or getting a second opinion) outside an insurance plan, but your primary lung cancer doctor needs to be covered by your policy unless cost is not an issue for you. Most insurance will allow you to get a second opinion outside your system, although they might not allow you to stay with that doctor.

- *Distance.* Certain types of treatment (e.g., chemotherapy and radiation) require multiple trips to the doctor or hospital. For some people, distance from the doctor will be a significant issue. Ask the hospital social worker about transportation alternatives or possibilities for inexpensive lodging. If you really like the doctor but are worried about the distance you will have to travel, particularly if you are feeling tired or sick, ask whether the oncologist and your primary doctor would be willing to work together. Some doctors feel very comfortable with this type of arrangement, while others do not.

- *Alternative medicine.* If you are interested in alternative medicine, you should address this issue during your first visit. It is crucial that both you and your doctor are comfortable discussing alternative medicine issues and that you are open with your doctor about any use of alternative medicine (see Question 61).

Because you are choosing a doctor who will be helping you to face life and death issues, the doctor's bedside manner, and your personal connection with him or her, are things to consider seriously. Trust and rapport are central to a strong doctor-patient relationship and should be given full consideration. Questions to consider:

Trust and rapport are central to a strong doctor-patient relationship and should be given full consideration.

- Does the doctor communicate in a clear and understandable manner? Is he or she willing to answer my questions? Is he or she a good listener or did he or she appear rushed?
- Does the doctor appear knowledgeable? Does the doctor inspire confidence?
- Does the doctor seem compassionate, caring, trustworthy?

- Did the doctor ask about me and my family—is he or she looking beyond my lung cancer?
- Does the doctor provide me options and explain them to me?

After your appointment or consultation, you should have a positive feeling that you and your doctor can work together as partners. If you are not comfortable with the first doctor you visit, you should not hesitate to look for another one.

On the other hand, you should remember that doctors are people, too. Although every patient would like to have a doctor who is a world-class, internationally known researcher with lots of time to spend with individual patients and has a wonderful bedside manner, this isn't always going to be possible. The bottom line is that you need to feel comfortable that your doctor knows what he or she is doing, is interested in you as an individual, and is willing to talk to you and answer your questions.

Finally, don't kill the messenger. Sometimes it is hard to separate the bad news from the person who has to give it. Just as it is not easy being on the receiving end of bad news, it is not easy being on the delivering end. Don't let your emotions about the diagnosis unfairly color your objective opinion of your doctor.

21. Should I get a second opinion?

The quality of your medical care is a critical factor in determining your chances for survival. A second opinion is an effective way to be sure you are getting the best

A second opinion is an effective way to be sure you are getting the best possible care and, at the same time, to gain peace of mind that you have explored all of your options.

possible care and, at the same time, to gain peace of mind that you have explored all of your options.

There are certain cases when a second opinion is particularly important:

- If you have been told that you are not a candidate for surgery but have reason to think you might be, you should seek another opinion from a thoracic surgeon. Surgery offers the best chance for a cure from lung cancer, and thoughts about who is a surgical candidate are changing. Thoracic surgeons who specialize in resecting lung cancers might be able to operate on some patients a general surgeon is not. Some patients become candidates for surgery after chemotherapy and/or radiation are used to shrink their tumors.

- If your doctor tells you that there is no treatment available for you, don't give up. It is rarely the case that there are no treatment options. A second opinion provides a different perspective and could bring additional choices for treatment.

- If your doctor seems reluctant to send your biopsy slides for mutational testing, you should enquire why. Is it because there is not enough material? Should you have another biopsy? Have they sent your slides for all of the most important, known mutations? These questions can sometimes be answered with a second opinion at a major medical center.

- If your doctor is associated with a small community hospital, it is a good idea to get a second opinion at a major cancer center or university hospital where research is performed, where the doctors might be more aware of the newest treatments, and where there could be additional clinical trial options for you.

- If you are uncomfortable with your doctor or have doubts about her recommendations for your care, you should look for another doctor. It is impossible to have a good doctor-patient relationship if you do not have confidence and trust in your doctor.

- If there is a question about your diagnosis (whether you have cancer, where it came from, or your tumor type), you should get a second pathology opinion (see Question 22). Errors in pathology are unusual but can occur. Your prognosis and treatment plan are determined by your pathological diagnosis, the diagnosis made by a pathologist after looking at your biopsy under a microscope. It is essential that your diagnosis is accurate.

Even when there is no compelling dilemma to resolve, a second opinion is often advisable. It can offer new options, confirm recommendations, or bring to light substandard care. If you get a conflicting second opinion, you can resolve issues by seeking a third opinion or by asking your primary care doctor (or another doctor) for guidance. Before seeking a second opinion, however, you should consider the potential downsides. The process of obtaining a second opinion can be emotionally draining, and will consume time and energy that you might not have. It can create confusion and delay treatment. You need to decide whether these negatives are offset by the potential long-term benefits of getting a second opinion.

Some patients worry that they will offend their doctor if they seek a second opinion. Keep in mind that you are entitled to seek a second opinion. Doctors are professionals who understand that patients will be seeking additional opinions or consultations. If you sense that your doctor is threatened by your intention to get a second opinion, then you might consider that to be further reason to pursue another perspective.

Unless you require emergency care, *you should try to get a second opinion before starting treatment.* This cannot be stressed enough. Once you have started treatment, it will be very difficult to switch to something else. Your doctor can advise you on how long you can afford to delay treatment. In the majority of cases, a few weeks won't make a difference to your health, and it makes sense to consider all options before making any treatment decision. There are also occasions after you have begun treatment when you might want to seek a second opinion; for example, if your disease is progressing and you are re-evaluating your treatment plan.

To make sure you get an independent assessment, it is a good idea to seek a second opinion from a doctor associated with a different institution than your original doctor. Many insurance companies will pay for second opinions, but it might be worth paying out of pocket for a second opinion from a particularly well-qualified specialist, even if he or she is outside your plan.

22. How do I go about getting a second opinion?

Arranging for a second opinion involves some logistics. You need to gather your medical records—including all reports and scans—to bring with you for a second opinion visit. We suggest hand-carrying them because outside records have a very bad habit of getting delayed (or lost) in the mail. Remember—if you have had X-rays or scans done in more than one place, you will need to go to each place to get them. The most important scans are your most recent CT scans and PET scan. Ask the person who gives them to you to double check to make sure they are in the package or on the disc. This cannot be overemphasized! Nothing is more frustrating than getting to the new doctor's office and finding out the most recent scans are not there, despite the fact you were assured they would be.

You also will need to get your pathology slides. A second pathology opinion is typically part of the second-opinion process. If you are satisfied with your care but would just like to confirm your pathology, this can be done easily without an office visit. The Joint Pathology Center is considered a leading pathology lab for second opinions (*www.jpc.capmed.mil*; (855) 393-3904).

23. How can I relate best to my doctor? What can I do to make my medical visits as productive as possible?

The doctor-patient relationship lies at the heart of patient care. This relationship will guide and support you throughout the course of your lung cancer. It is your job, and your doctor's, to nurture this relationship and to work toward a partnership based on mutual trust and respect. Although difficulties between doctor and patient can occur at times, just as they do in any relationship, these problems will be minimized if good communication is maintained. Remember that your doctor is not a mind reader. It is your responsibility to be open and honest and to bring up any concerns, needs or preferences you might have. It is especially important that you feel comfortable discussing sensitive issues, such as your use of alternative medicine treatments, your lifestyle (smoking, drinking, drugs), end-of-life issues, and sexual concerns. Keep in mind that conversations between doctor and patient are confidential (your family does not need to know if you don't want them to) and

It is your responsibility to be open and honest and to bring up any concerns, needs or preferences you might have.

that the more your doctor knows about issues that could impact your health, the better care you will receive.

At your first visit you should address the issues of how much information you want from your doctor and how involved you would like to be in the decisions that are made about your care. Some patients want to know everything about their condition, and they want to make all the decisions themselves. Some patients find too much information anxiety-provoking. These patients would prefer to hear less information (or only the good news) and are more comfortable allowing their doctor to make all the decisions. Many patients fall somewhere in between. Whatever your preferences might be, and they can change over time, you need to communicate them to your doctor. If you feel that your doctor is not responsive to your needs, or if you have other concerns regarding your relationship, you should bring them up before they reach a crisis stage. If you and your doctor cannot resolve disagreements in a productive and satisfactory manner, you should look for another doctor.

It is also important to discuss with your doctor how much you do or do not want your family involved. If you do not want your doctor discussing your case with family members without you present, tell your doctor. Most doctors will ask you to sign a release of information form, giving them permission to talk to whomever you designate, before they will talk to a friend or family member when you are not around.

Think about what you are going to say to your doctor ahead of time. Remember, he or she has a certain amount of time to spend with you. Before your appointment consider which concerns are most pressing and write them down in order of importance. This tactic will help you focus and make the most effective use of the limited time you have with your doctor. Too often, patients spend their time with the doctor trying to remember if the pain started on Monday when Aunt Ellie was visiting for dinner, or on Tuesday afternoon when they went out shopping, or Tuesday morning before breakfast, or maybe Wednesday when Aunt Ellie came back to pick up the casserole dish she forgot. If you choose to review events in great detail, you risk running out of the time that your doctor has for addressing more important issues.

If you have symptoms to report, describe them clearly and concisely. Be prepared to answer your doctor's questions, such as when the symptoms started, how often they occur, and how long they last. In most instances, you do not have to be exact; saying "early last week" or "about 2 months ago" will suffice. Don't be afraid to mention the emotional and social issues that are affecting you, in addition to any physical problems you have.

Always bring someone with you to your appointment. It is impossible to remember all that is said during an office visit, and emotions can cloud what a patient hears. It helps to have someone else along who can write down what the doctor says. Tape recording your conversations are another very helpful way of remembering exactly what transpired. As long as you tell the doctor what you are doing, most physicians have no problem with this. It is important that you understand everything that your doctor tells you. If something is unclear, say so, and ask questions until you are satisfied that you understand completely.

Many oncologists have an oncology nurse, nurse practitioner, or patient navigator with whom they work closely.

Get this person's name and number! He or she can answer a lot of questions the doctor might not have time for, particularly between visits, and is often your patient advocate with your doctor. In many cases, he or she will be the go-between between you and your doctor, particularly between visits when problems or questions come up.

Be sure that all necessary tests are completed prior to your visit and that you have all the information you need. This includes having the required referrals, if any, and a current list of the prescription and nonprescription drugs you are taking. (It is very helpful to *bring the actual pill bottles along with EACH visit.*) Bring a notebook or binder that contains your medical information and paperwork to each appointment. If you can present your doctor with the information she needs to care for you in an efficient and clear manner, you will go a long way toward increasing the quality of your relationship with your doctor and, ultimately, the quality of your care.

Coping with Your Diagnosis

What is my prognosis? Can I survive lung cancer?

How do I manage my emotions? Should I seek professional counseling? What types of psychosocial support are available to me?

How do I regain control of my life after my lung cancer diagnosis? How do I get past the emotional impact and move forward?

More . . .

24. What is my prognosis? Can I survive lung cancer?

It is natural to worry about what a lung cancer diagnosis will mean for you and your family and to wonder whether you will die from your cancer. Most patients want to know their prognosis so that they can plan for the future and prepare for what lies ahead. Your prognosis is a prediction of how well you will do and how long you will live. Your prognosis is influenced by many factors, including the type of lung cancer you have, how far your cancer has spread, how aggressive your tumor is, your age, and your general health. The treatment you receive could affect your prognosis, and your prognosis might change over time. The best person to discuss your prognosis with is your doctor.

To arrive at your prognosis, your doctor will take into consideration the lung cancer statistics, his or her experience with other lung cancer patients, and what he or she knows about your individual case.

To arrive at your prognosis, your doctor will take into consideration the lung cancer statistics, his or her experience with other lung cancer patients, and what he or she knows about your individual case. It is important to remember that your prognosis is only an educated guess and that it is impossible for anyone, even your doctor, to predict your future with certainty.

You can become familiar with the survival statistics for lung cancer through discussions with your doctor or from other sources. For lung cancer patients, survival rates are not encouraging, and it can be overwhelming to learn about them. It is helpful to understand why these statistics might not be accurate for you. Survival statistics, like those compiled by the American Cancer Society, usually measure the 5-year survival of a group of patients with similar characteristics. These statistics are averages and do not represent the prognosis for any given individual. Your unique characteristics will cause your prognosis to differ from the average lung cancer patient. You should also be aware that the survival statistics reflect the outcomes of patients who were treated with older therapies. They don't take into account the newer, more effective treatments that are available today or the promising treatments that will be available in the near future.

Although it makes sense to plan for every eventuality when you are facing a potentially deadly disease, you should not allow statistics or a bleak prediction by your doctor to dictate your future. There are patients who have survived every stage of lung cancer and patients who have outlived their doctors' predictions. Your prognosis provides a perspective, but it is not etched in stone. Try to focus your thoughts on the tens of thousands of people who have survived lung cancer. There is no reason why you can't be one of them.

While it is good to hope for the best, you should also prepare for the worst. Now is a good time to assess your personal, financial, and legal affairs (see Questions 30 and 96). Working on these issues while you are undergoing treatment in no way means you are giving up. It could, however, relieve you of other worries down the road.

COPING WITH YOUR DIAGNOSIS

EMOTIONAL ASPECTS

25. How do I manage my emotions? Should I seek professional counseling? What types of psychosocial support are available to me?

A lung cancer diagnosis brings with it a tidal wave of emotions and a sense of uncertainty about the future. Feelings of shock, denial, anger, fear, helplessness, sadness, and anxiety are all normal responses to a life-threatening crisis. You likely will experience a range of emotions that will fluctuate from moment to moment and vary over the course of your disease. It is important to remember that there is no right or wrong way to feel and that it can take time to learn to cope with your emotions. You might hear from others that you can influence your chances for survival through positive thinking and an upbeat attitude. Although this approach might be helpful to you, you should not worry that feelings of anger or sadness will cause your tumor to grow faster—this is a common worry among cancer patients, but there is no evidence that it occurs. Expressing your emotions, both positive and negative, can be an effective way to relieve stress. You should feel comfortable using whatever coping mechanisms work for you and not be concerned about being a perfect cancer patient.

One method of coping that works well for many cancer patients is to reach out to others for emotional support. Spending time with family, friends, neighbors, and members of your religious community could help to reduce the sense of isolation brought on by your cancer diagnosis. In particular, connecting with other lung cancer survivors can be heartening and inspiring. People who are facing similar challenges share common concerns, experiences, and hopes for the future. The National Lung Cancer Partnership (*www.NationalLungCancerPartnership.org*) provides educational materials and resources for those dealing with a diagnosis of lung cancer. The Lung Cancer Alliance (LCA) provides a phone buddy program that will pair you with someone who has a similar type and stage of lung cancer.

LCA also maintains a geographic listing of in-person lung cancer support groups. Support groups are not for everyone, but if you are looking for a community of people who will know exactly how you feel and can offer emotional support and practical information, a lung cancer support group will likely meet your needs. If no group is available in your area or if you are reticent to participate in an in-person group, you might consider joining an online support group (also called a discussion list or a mailing list). The Association for Cancer Online Resources (ACOR) maintains four lung cancer lists: a general list (LUNG-ONC), and specific lists for small cell lung cancer (LUNG-SCLC), non-small cell lung cancer (LUNG-NSCLC), and bronchioloalveolar carcinoma (LUNG-AIS). Online support groups are especially valuable for patients who are physically unable to attend in-person groups but who wish to participate in a lung cancer community. (See Question 100 for information about locating lung cancer support groups.)

If you find that your distress persists and that you are having ongoing difficulty managing your emotions, you might want to seek mental health, social work, or pastoral counseling. Your doctor can refer you to a psychiatrist or psychologist who can evaluate your symptoms and provide therapy to help relieve your distress. Clinical

If you find that your distress persists and that you are having ongoing difficulty managing your emotions, you might want to seek mental health, social work, or pastoral counseling.

social workers can also provide counseling and can alert you to other sources of support. Mental health professionals can teach you coping strategies, such as relaxation techniques and guided imagery. Your religion can provide comfort at this time, and you might want to approach your clergy about spiritual counseling.

26. How do I regain control of my life after my lung cancer diagnosis? How do I get past the emotional impact and move forward?

A lung cancer diagnosis can be overwhelming, making it difficult to absorb information and focus on what needs to be done. Your mind might be clouded with thoughts and worries about what your lung cancer will mean for you and your family. To move forward effectively, you need to make a mental adjustment. You need to redirect your energies toward the things you can control. Although you cannot change the fact that you have lung cancer, you can control how you respond to this challenge.

A first step toward gaining control of your thoughts is to realize that you are not alone in facing lung cancer.

A first step toward gaining control of your thoughts is to realize that you are not alone in facing lung cancer. Thousands of people are surviving with lung cancer and leading happy, productive lives. The National Coalition for Cancer Survivorship defines a cancer survivor as anyone with a diagnosis of cancer, and you are considered a survivor from the moment of diagnosis. Cancer is not a death sentence. Many people view cancer as a chronic disease, something to be treated and managed. Keeping this concept in mind will help make your cancer experience less frightening.

Your new job is to become an involved cancer patient. The process of taking an active role in your health care will help you to gain stability, confidence, and hope. Your efforts can make a difference in the quality of your care.

Try to focus your energies on the following activities:

- *Adopting a healthy lifestyle.* Not smoking, maintaining adequate nutrition, and minimizing stress can all help your ability to fight your disease and withstand the effects of your cancer treatment (see Part 9).

- *Assembling a medical team.* You need to find doctors who you can trust and who will provide you with excellent care. This could involve getting second opinions. You should keep in mind that good communication with all members of your medical team—including support personnel—is critical to the quality of care you receive (see Question 19).

- *Gathering information and making informed decisions.* You need to learn all you can about lung cancer and its treatment so that you will understand what is happening to you. After gathering information and discussing your treatment options with your doctor, you will be able to make informed decisions about your care.

- *Learning to navigate the healthcare system.* Your doctor's office staff and hospital social workers can help you learn how to navigate the healthcare system. This will make your appointments more productive and minimize the aggravation over medical paperwork, insurance, and financial concerns (see Questions 30 and 31).

Consider joining a patient advocacy group. There are several specific to lung cancer and you can research the various groups to find one whose mission best fits your interest. For example, you might try research, fundraising, patient support, education/awareness, or legislative initiatives (see Question 100).

27. How do I cope with the stigma of having a self-inflicted disease? Should I feel guilty about my smoking? What if I never smoked—how do I cope with having a smoker's disease?

Your emotions following your lung cancer diagnosis are likely to be complicated by your feelings about smoking. If you were an active smoker, you might experience feelings of guilt. If you never smoked, or if you had stopped smoking years before, you might be shocked that you have been diagnosed with a smoking-related disease. This personal conflict over smoking is often made worse by the reactions of those around you and by the lack of public support for people with lung cancer. Some family members and friends could be angry with you for having caused your own disease. When acquaintances learn of your lung cancer, you could get tired of hearing the inevitable question, "Did you smoke?" And it is devastating to discover that the support services, media coverage, and fundraising events that are routine for other major cancers are less common for lung cancer. This lack of public empathy and support is demoralizing and adds additional stress to the challenges you face. Thankfully, there are now several organizations, such as the National Lung Cancer Partnership, working very hard to raise awareness and educate the general public about the realities of lung cancer, as well as to raise research funds.

It is important to let go of any feelings of guilt. Guilt over smoking wastes energy that could go toward fighting your disease. Keep in mind that smoking is legal (you have done nothing wrong) and is highly addicting. More than 90% of smokers begin smoking as teenagers, at an age when they are rebellious, feel invulnerable, and are unlikely to believe or understand the risks and addictive nature of tobacco. The tobacco companies continue to play an unconscionable role in perpetuating this deadly addiction among young people. In addition, they have specifically manufactured their cigarettes to be highly physically addictive.

It is also important to note that the majority of lung cancer diagnoses occur in a combination of former smokers (50%) and those who have never smoked (15%–20%). Regardless of whether one has or hasn't smoked, no one deserves lung cancer.

Charles adds ...

"I believe people link lung cancer to smoking, at least in part, as a way of convincing themselves that it could never happen to them—only smokers have to be concerned about having this killer disease. It is that attitude of it can't happen to me that has affected interest, concern, and funding. Ignorance is not bliss; it can be fatal. As a never-smoker who has had lung cancer, I have learned that lung cancer is a human disease, not just a smoker's disease."

One productive step you can take to help de-stigmatize this disease is to use whatever opportunities you have to put a face on lung cancer. Do not be afraid to speak up and identify yourself as a lung cancer survivor. The public needs to know that lung cancer affects everyone—mothers, fathers, sisters, brothers, and loved ones, young and old. It is easy to ignore lung cancer

It is important to let go of any feelings of guilt. Guilt over smoking wastes energy that could go toward fighting your disease.

COPING WITH YOUR DIAGNOSIS

when smokers are cited as its victims. A smoker is an abstract notion, not a person with a life-threatening disease, worthy of caring and support. People with lung cancer are good people too—they have names, faces, and families—and they deserve the same respect afforded other cancer survivors. You can also advocate through an established organization that is dedicated to changing the perception about lung cancer (see Question 26). For some, advocacy efforts can help the patient and/or family members focus emotional energy in a positive and hopeful way.

Tomma adds...

"Now that I have been a survivor of Stage IIIB and an advocate for lung cancer awareness for more than 5 years, I have learned some ways to deal with the guilt and the stigma. It isn't easy to look someone in the eye and admit that I had been a smoker at one time, but I now realize that many other medical conditions such as heart disease are caused by bad habits. We just don't play the blame game with that. Once we learn the statistics about lung cancer patients, we realize that it can't be and isn't just about smoking and this so-called self-inflicted disease."

28. What should I tell my children about my lung cancer? What if my children are grown?

Lung cancer does not just affect patients; it also affects their families and friends. Children are particularly vulnerable, and their welfare is often the primary concern of parents with lung cancer. Children should be told about a parent's illness. If things are hidden from them, or they are lied to, they will at some point sense that something is wrong. This might cause them to feel isolated or to fear that things are worse than they are. There is a good chance they will discover the truth anyway—either from overhearing conversations or from an unintentional slip—causing a loss of trust between parent and child at a time when that trust is so vital. It is better if they hear the news directly from a parent, so that it can be presented in a controlled and reassuring manner. In general, learning the truth about a parent's cancer will reduce a child's fear, even if the truth is frightening. It will remove uncertainty and enable the child to learn productive ways of coping with a difficult situation.

Before discussing your lung cancer with your child, you should give what you are going to say some thought, and try to anticipate questions your child might ask.

Consider the following:

- *Children need information presented in a clear, understandable manner.* Appropriate information will depend on the age and emotional maturity of the child. You know your child best. In general, you do not need to tell your child every detail, but you should not lie. You can be honest about uncertainty, but try to present the information in a realistic, yet hopeful, light.

- *Prepare your child for what will happen next.* If your child knows ahead of time that you will be having treatment and that you will experience side effects from your treatment (such as losing your hair or being very tired), he or she will be better able to adjust to your condition. It is helpful to stress that these effects are temporary.

- *Reassure your child that someone will always be there to take care of him.* Your child might worry about how your cancer will impact his or her life. It is important that your child's environment and activities be kept as normal as possible.

- *Encourage your child to express his feelings and to ask questions.* You might want to provide opportunities for your child to express his thoughts in writing or by drawing pictures.

- *Let your child know that he or she might hear some frightening things about cancer but that he should come to you to get the facts.* You can tell him that while some people die from cancer, many people survive because they get effective treatments from their doctors. Stress that your doctors are taking good care of you and that you are getting the best treatments.

- *Your child might want to meet your doctor.* This can be a very positive experience. It can allow a child to feel more involved and to gain a more concrete understanding of what is being done to make you better. It is important that you take your cue about this from your child. No child should be forced to participate in anything beyond his or her comfort level.

- *Let your child know that he or she did nothing to cause your cancer.* If you smoked, you might anticipate a question about whether you caused your lung cancer by smoking.

It is a good idea to let your child's teachers (and the school psychologist, social worker, and/or guidance counselor) know about your lung cancer and family situation.

It is a good idea to let your child's teachers (and the school psychologist, social worker, and/or guidance counselor) know about your lung cancer and family situation. These professionals can be extremely supportive during this time and can be alert to signs that your child might need extra help to cope with his or her feelings about your cancer. Be aware that older children need as much support as younger children do, and efforts should take into account the way your child expresses herself or himself in times of distress.

Sandy adds...

"Since my son's birth, he has given me a whole new meaning for living. I couldn't bear the thought of missing him grow up or him growing up without his mommy. We kept it very basic trying to explain the things he would see, like possible hair loss from chemo, lower energy level, and mommy in the hospital when part of her lung was removed. He was too young to understand the severity of the situation, which gave me comfort. I needed to maintain as normal a day-to-day life as possible. We were always honest with him even through the hard questions."

If you have adult children, what you choose to share with them about your lung cancer will depend upon the nature of your relationship. You will likely find that your children will react as you would have expected, but do not be surprised if your cancer causes them to act in ways you might not have anticipated. Even as an adult, it can be overwhelming to learn that one's parent has a life-threatening illness. If you find your children acting in ways that hurt you or make you uncomfortable (such as being overprotective or becoming emotionally distant), try to express your feelings and keep the lines of communication open. This becomes especially critical when your children do not live close to you, as is often the case with grown children. In particular, you will need to work out a system for relaying important medical information. You could feel comfortable handling this yourself, or you might have the person who accompanies you to doctor visits talk to your children about medical details. In any case, you should let your doctor know which family members you would like to be involved in your care.

Sandy adds...

"Now 15 years old, [my son] recently surprised me when reflecting on the time when I was sick and said, 'I'm really glad I was too young to understand what was happening to you.' I was too but shared that I knew he would be able to handle anything life has in store for him."

29. What do caregivers need to know to best support a person with lung cancer?

Caregivers play a vital role in the life of lung cancer patients, but they shoulder responsibilities that can be overwhelming at times. Demands placed on caregivers can be both emotionally and physically exhausting. To effectively support patients, caregivers must attend to their own needs, just as they attend to the needs of their patients. The following suggestions will help you to minimize the stress of the caregiving experience and become a more effective caregiver.

- *Educate yourself about lung cancer.* Learn as much as you can about lung cancer, its treatments and side effects, and disease complications such as breathing distress. This will help you to understand what the patient is going through and allow you to be a better cancer supporter and advocate. Advocacy organizations and online resources can be very helpful (see the Appendix).

- *Establish a relationship with the patient's doctor.* The patient should let his doctor know that you are the primary caregiver. With the patient's permission, the doctor will answer any questions you have. Be sure you understand your specific responsibilities for care at home (such as dispensing medication, monitoring and reporting symptoms, and managing IV and oxygen therapy) and under what circumstances you should call the doctor's office for assistance.

- *Seek out help for daily tasks.* Don't try to go it alone. Let family and friends know the work involved in being a caregiver, and identify specific ways that they might help you, such as running errands or spending time with the patient so you can take a break. If you can delegate responsibility for managing insurance paperwork to a trusted and competent person, this will relieve you of a significant source of aggravation.

- *Monitor your stress and health.* Be mindful of how you are feeling, and try to address issues before you become overwhelmed. Set limits for what you can do and be sure to take time away from the patient to attend to your own needs. Remember that caring for yourself is as important as caring for your loved one. If you are not healthy, the patient will suffer, too.

- *Keep communication open.* Providing emotional support is a critical aspect of care giving. Often just listening is enough. You can and should talk about your own feelings and fears about the future. If you have anger over the patient's previous or current smoking, this is not a productive time to vent. The patient needs your unconditional support. It can be useful to discuss the changes in your relationship that have come about as a result of the patient's lung cancer diagnosis.

- *Seek out emotional support.* Find people you can talk to about your experiences. This can be good friends or other family members. It is particularly helpful to find other caregivers who share your perspective and experience. You can often find support groups for caregivers and family members at hospitals and through organizations like CancerCare and the Wellness Community. The Association of Cancer

Online Resources (ACOR) has an online support group for caregivers of people with cancer. (For further information on these resources, see the Support Services section of the Appendix.) If you have persistent difficulties coping with your situation, you should seek professional counseling.

- *Focus on the positive.* Although the challenges of care giving are often daunting, the rewards are immeasurable. Care giving is the greatest gift that one can give to a cancer patient. You gain the satisfaction of knowing that you actively helped your loved one in a time of need. Amidst the tedium, the aggravation, and the anguish are moments of tenderness and love that would not exist outside the cancer experience. If your loved one has limited time, you gain peace of mind that you have done the best you could to help him through his most difficult journey.

PRACTICAL ASPECTS

As difficult as it is to think about, newly diagnosed cancer patients must pay immediate and careful attention to insurance and financial concerns.

30. What insurance and financial concerns do I need to address following a lung cancer diagnosis?

As difficult as it is to think about, newly diagnosed cancer patients must pay immediate and careful attention to insurance and financial concerns. The costs associated with cancer care can present an enormous economic burden. For the uninsured and underinsured, this financial strain can be devastating. Even for those who are well insured, cancer-related medical expenses can cause financial hardship. Inadequate insurance and insufficient finances can have a negative impact on the amount and quality of your cancer care and on the course of your disease. Being proactive about your financial needs can help you minimize the cost and aggravation associated with your cancer experience and will ensure that you can afford quality health care.

Your first step should be to examine your current health insurance coverage. Familiarize yourself with your policy and learn the scope of your medical coverage. What are your benefits? What are your restrictions? Are there circumstances under which you need pre-certification for coverage? Most physicians and/or hospitals have financial counselors who can advise you as to what the treatments will cost and what your cost or responsibility will be.

Look at the sections on how to file claims and how to appeal denied claims. Try to anticipate what your medical needs might be, including the possibility for long-term care or **hospice**. Do you have adequate coverage in your current policy? If you do not have insurance or are underinsured, there are still options available to you despite your cancer diagnosis.

After assessing your insurance coverage, you need to examine your financial resources. Will you be able to comfortably pay all out-of-pocket costs? There are costs associated with cancer beyond health care, such as additional transportation and childcare expenses. You must also be prepared for the possibility that you might not be able to work for an indefinite period of time. Depending on your situation, you might need to convert your life insurance policy, retirement account, or other personal property into liquid assets. Now is the time to explore all potential avenues for financial assistance. You should get sound advice, and give careful consideration, before making any financial decisions. A financial counselor is

Hospice

An organization that provides end-of-life care that focuses on palliative rather than curative care and provides a wide range of support to dying patients and their families.

best able to advise you on your current and future financial health.

There is a wide range of resources that you can turn to for assistance with your insurance and financial needs. Some of these resources include your doctor's staff, your hospital's social worker or financial counselor, your employer's benefits manager, and nonprofit organizations such as the American Cancer Society, United Way, CancerCare, and the Patient Advocate Foundation. These individuals and organizations can help you to navigate the complex insurance and managed care systems, provide direct assistance with your paperwork or finances, or refer you to additional sources of support in your community. They can lead you to services and programs, both private and government-sponsored, that you might be eligible for and that could be useful to you.

Some of these could include:

- Additional health insurance through private carriers or government entitlement programs, such as Medicare and Medicaid
- Disability benefits (private, employment, state, social security)
- Legal protections for getting and retaining health insurance coverage, preventing gaps in coverage, and for when you have been discriminated against due to your lung cancer
- Allowable medical deductions on your income taxes
- Family Medical Leave Act (FMLA)
- Veterans' Benefits
- Specialized assistance programs for patients who require transportation for cancer care or access to free medications

For further information on these organizations, services, and government programs, see the Appendix. For an outstanding book that provides comprehensive, in-depth information on this subject, see David S. Landry's *Be Prepared: The Complete Financial, Legal, and Practical Guide to Living with Cancer, HIV, and Other Life-Challenging Conditions.*

31. How do I learn to manage the medical paperwork? What are medical records, and what should I know about them?

Lung cancer generates a seemingly endless stream of medical appointments and paperwork. Handling the administrative tasks associated with your cancer care takes up substantial amounts of time and adds further stress to your already difficult situation. By understanding and organizing your medical information and paperwork, you will be better equipped to manage the logistics of your cancer care. This will help save you valuable time and reduce your aggravation.

Health information generated about you by your healthcare providers and your medical facilities becomes part of your medical record. Chart notes kept by your doctor, lab tests, CT scan reports, pathology reports, consultation reports, and hospital discharge notes are all examples of medical records. Medical records are used by your providers to plan your care and to communicate with each other. They are also used by insurance companies and legal entities to document your health care. Accurate health information compiled in a timely manner is essential for quality health care. Because mistakes are not uncommon, you should obtain copies of your medical reports at the time they are generated. Copies of chart notes are usually required when applying for social security benefits. In most cases, healthcare providers and medical facilities will accommodate patient requests for copies of medical records, although they might charge a small fee. (State laws vary on patient access to medical records. You can contact your state's health department to determine your rights.) The confidentiality of your personal health information (PHI) is protected by law. Your medical records will not be shared with third parties without your authorization.

An effective way to manage the medical information and records that you will acquire during the course of your care is to use a three-ring binder with multiple dividers. This method of organization can be tailored to your needs, and the binder can be brought with you to every medical appointment. Binder sections might include personal information, medical information (including staging and treatment details), names of healthcare providers, reports (imaging, consultation, lab), pre-testing instructions, a summary of your treatments and medications, and insurance and billing records.

In addition to paper records, you need to collect copies of your imaging films, such as X-rays and CT scans. This is best done at the time of the study. Be sure to tell the technician prior to your scan that you would like duplicate copies of the films to bring home with you. In most instances, this request is easily accommodated. In some cases, you could have a delay in getting films (from a couple of hours to a day), and you might have to pay a small fee. If they give you the actual films, they can be kept in an inexpensive portfolio, which you can purchase at any art supply store. More and more often, however, they are given to you on a computer disk or CD. Unfortunately, these tend to get lost easily. Ask if you can have a second copy made for yourself.

You might also need to get your pathology slides. These slides contain tissue specimens from your biopsy or surgery. You will need these slides when you are obtaining a second opinion. You can arrange with the hospital tissue bank or your doctor's office to obtain these yourself or to have them sent directly to the consulting physician. It is helpful to know that the tissue bank also has your tumor block, which is an amount of your tissue left over from the operation that is generally kept for a number of years (this varies by institution) because there could be occasions when you need additional tissue specimens for further testing.

What Types of Treatments Are Available for Lung Cancer?

What are the goals of treatment?

What are the different types of surgeries used for treating lung cancer? How are they performed?

What does my surgeon mean when he or she says, "I got it all"? Does this mean I am cured?

More . . .

32. What types of treatments are available for lung cancer?

Radiotherapy

The treatment of disease with ionizing radiation. Also called radiation therapy.

Intravenous

In the vein.

Targeted therapy

Therapy directed at aspects of the cell that are specific for cancer.

The three traditional treatments for lung cancer include surgery, radiation therapy, and chemotherapy. Lung surgery commonly involves an operation to remove the tumor, along with nearby lymph nodes (see Question 35). Radiation therapy (or **radiotherapy**) is the delivery of a beam of radiation aimed at the tumor with the goal of killing some or all of the cancer cells, thus shrinking the tumor (see Question 47). Both surgery and radiotherapy are local forms of treatment, which means that they kill or remove only the tumor they are aimed at. Chemotherapy is a word for medications that kill cancer cells or stop their growth (see Question 40). Most chemotherapies are given **intravenously** (injected or dripped into the veins), but some are pills and are given orally. In either case, they get into the bloodstream and circulate around the body. Because blood flows through all parts of the body, in theory, cancer cells anywhere in the body would be exposed to the chemotherapy. Therefore, chemotherapy is a systemic therapy. Recently, **targeted therapy** has been added as a fourth modality for lung cancer. Targeted therapies are oral or intravenous medications that target abnormalities found in tumors or cancer cells but not normal tissues. Although targeted therapies are systemic treatments, like chemotherapy, they tend to have fewer side effects because they do not affect normal cells. Some examples of targeted therapies include bevacizumab (Avastin), erlotinib (Tarceva), and crizotinib (Xalkori).

New treatments for lung cancer are always being tested in research studies known as clinical trials. You should familiarize yourself with the advantages and disadvantages of participation in clinical trials and explore the treatment options available to you through clinical trials (see Questions 59 and 60). If you are considering alternative therapies, such as herbal therapies, you should have an understanding of how to evaluate them. Alternative therapies are treatments not endorsed by the traditional medical establishment because their effectiveness and safety have not been proven in rigorous scientific studies (see Question 61).

33. What are the goals of treatment?

For patients with early stage (Stage I–IIIA) cancer, the goals of treatment are usually cure. **Curative treatment** is just what it sounds like—treatment given in order to cure the patient of his or her cancer. Typically, curative treatment for non-small cell lung cancer will include surgery if the disease was discovered at an early stage. For Stage III disease (see Question 57), curative treatment could consist of chemotherapy and surgery or chemotherapy and radiation therapy. For a limited-stage small cell lung cancer, curative treatment usually consists of a combination of both chemotherapy and radiation therapy to the tumor in the chest.

Curative treatment

Treatment given with the intent to cure the patient of his or her cancer.

Realistically, treatment of advanced, metastatic lung cancer is usually not curative. Instead, the goals of treatment are to prolong survival, shrink the tumor if at all possible, improve the symptoms from the tumor, and all the while maintain a good quality of life. Chemotherapy is administered with the intent to shrink the tumor or at least keep it stable and stop it from growing. In doing so, one hopes to prolong life and decrease symptoms, thereby improving quality of life.

The general sense of well-being of the patient is an important prognostic factor; that is, patients who have relatively few symptoms are more likely to do well than patients who are very fatigued, weak, anorexic, and losing weight.

Palliation usually refers to treatments that are directed at reducing symptoms. Radiation therapy is an example of a treatment that can be either curative or palliative. Sometimes, high doses of radiation therapy can be administered with curative intent to lung cancer patients with local disease who are not candidates for surgery. More commonly, however, somewhat lower doses of radiation therapy (palliative doses) are administered to shrink a tumor that is causing symptoms, such as metastases that have spread to the brain, spinal cord, and bone. Occasionally, it is also given to the primary tumor in the chest. Palliative radiation is usually effective at reducing the neurological signs and symptoms from the brain metastasis; reducing pain from the bone metastasis and preventing bone fractures; and improving tumor-related symptoms, such as shortness of breath, cough, or bleeding.

It is appropriate to ask your doctor about the goals of treatment if he or she has not already told you.

34. What is performance status, and why is it important?

Performance status is a term used to describe the general condition of the patient. The general sense of well-being of the patient is an important prognostic factor; that is, patients who have relatively few symptoms are more likely to do better than patients who are very fatigued, weak, anorexic, and losing weight. Several different grading systems for performance status are currently used, including the ECOG (Eastern Cooperative Oncology Group) grading system and the Zubrich or Karnofsky grading system. The ECOG grading system is rated on a scale of 0 to 4 and is defined in **Table 2**. This grading system is defined on a scale of 100% to 0%, where 100% is totally **asymptomatic**, and 0% is very near death.

Table 2 ECOG PS Grading System

PS	GRADE DESCRIPTION
0	Totally asymptomatic
1	Mildly symptomatic, able to perform daily activities
2	Able to perform daily activities with assistance, spends less than 50% of the day in bed
3	Needs considerable assistance for performing daily activities, spends greater than 50% of the day in bed
4	Totally bedridden, unable to care for oneself

Performance status is often used in defining eligibility for a clinical trial (see Question 59). Because patients with poor performance status are often very weak, most clinical trials exclude patients with a performance status of 2 through 4. There is, however, increasing interest in defining treatment for these patients as well.

SURGERY

35. What are the different types of surgeries used for treating lung cancer? How are they performed?

Ideally, surgery for lung cancer should be done by a thoracic surgeon (see Questions 19 and 35). The type of surgery performed depends upon the stage of tumor, and the medical condition of the patient. The most typical operation is a lobectomy and mediastinal **lymph node dissection**. A **lobectomy** is the removal of the lobe of the lung in which the tumor is located. A mediastinal lymph node dissection consists of removing some or all of the mediastinal lymph nodes (the lymph nodes

Lymph node dissection

Surgical removal of lymph nodes.

Lobectomy

Surgical removal of a lobe of the lung.

between the lung and heart). This is often done to determine whether the tumor has spread to these lymph nodes. Occasionally, a patient might be unable to tolerate a lobectomy because underlying bronchitis or emphysema (COPD) makes it too difficult for the remaining lung to keep the person alive. In these cases, a surgeon will sometimes do a **wedge resection**. This consists of removing the tumor and a small amount of lung tissue surrounding the tumor, but not the whole lobe. A wedge resection will preserve more normal lung, but the chances of the cancer coming back are somewhat higher.

Occasionally, the tumor is located in an area such that all the lobes of the lung on that side are involved, meaning that they all contain some tumor. Sometimes the tumor is located in the largest airway on that side (the right or left main stem bronchus, which is the first major division of the trachea, the air pipe that delivers air to the lungs). If one of the main stem bronchi is involved, or if the tumor involves all the lobes on one side, a **pneumonectomy** must be performed. In a pneumonectomy, the whole lung is removed. Obviously, this is a much bigger procedure than a lobectomy or a wedge resection. Although a person with two normal lungs should be able to tolerate removal of one of the lungs without a major impact on his or her breathing, very often patients who have been smoking and have a substantial amount of emphysema or bronchitis are not able to tolerate a pneumonectomy.

Typically, lung surgery involves an operation called a **thoracotomy**, which requires the surgeon to make a large incision in the chest to gain access to the lungs. Video assisted thoracoscopic surgery (VATS) is an example of a less invasive surgical technique (also called **minimally invasive surgery**), which involves smaller

Wedge resection

Surgical removal of the tumor and a small amount of lung tissue surrounding the tumor.

Pneumonectomy

Surgical removal of the entire lung.

Thoracotomy

A common type of lung surgery that requires a large incision to provide access to the lungs.

Minimally invasive surgery

Surgery which uses smaller incisions than a regular operation and thus is less painful for the patient post-operatively. In order to be able to operate through such a small incision, the surgeon must used advanced, fibro electronic instruments.

incisions and therefore reduced post-operative pain and complications and shorter hospital stays. Robotic surgery is another form of minimally invasive surgery, in which the surgeon manipulates the instruments via a computer screen.

36. What determines whether I am able to have surgery?

To determine whether a patient is a candidate for surgery, three things must be established first:

1. Has the cancer metastasized? If the cancer has spread to other organs (Stage IV), a surgical cure is not possible and it does not make sense to do a large operation, considering the side effects, cost, and risks associated with surgery. Therefore, patients with metastatic disease usually do not undergo a curative resection.

2. The tumor must be **resectable**—that is, located in a place that the surgeon will be able to get to and completely remove. For example, if the tumor involves the heart, the surgeon obviously cannot safely remove the heart, and the tumor would be considered unresectable. In general, a tumor is considered unresectable if it involves any other major structures in the center of the chest, such as the heart, the large blood vessels going in and out of the heart, or the windpipe leading from the mouth to the lungs (the trachea).

3. The third criterion for surgery is that a patient must be healthy enough to withstand it. In particular, this involves two organs—the heart and the lungs.

Resectable

Able to be surgically removed (resected).

71

a. If you have a history of heart disease, such as congestive heart failure, angina, or heart attacks, your surgeon will want to make sure that it is safe to operate on you, so that the stress of the surgery will not result in a heart attack. He or she might ask you to see a cardiologist, or heart doctor. The cardiologist will take a history, examine you, and might order an EKG, echo-cardiogram, or stress test before giving a final recommendation.

b. Many patients with lung cancer are smokers or former smokers and have some degree of emphysema or bronchitis (also known as chronic obstructive pulmonary disease, or COPD). If your doctor suspects you have COPD, he or she will order **pulmonary function tests** (PFTs). PFTs are a series of breathing tests that can help determine how healthy your lungs are and whether your remaining lungs will be able to support you if a portion of one of them has been removed. Your doctor might also order a preoperative quantitative perfusion scan, which is a nuclear medicine scan designed to predict how much lung function you will be left with after the operation.

Pulmonary function tests (PFTs)

A group of breathing tests used to determine lung health.

37. What can I expect before surgery, and what can I do to prepare for it?

If you are a current smoker, the most important thing you can do to prepare for surgery is stop smoking. Regardless of whether you decide to quit permanently, stopping even if only for a few days or weeks in advance will markedly improve your ability to tolerate the operation. This cannot be stressed enough. Many thoracic

If you are a current smoker, the most important thing you can do to prepare for surgery is stop smoking.

surgeons will not operate on a patient who is still actively smoking because of the higher risks associated with the surgery. There are a number of techniques and medications approved to help people stop smoking. Ask your doctor if you need help, including a referral to a smoking cessation clinic.

Prior to the operation, your surgeon will explain the procedure to you and arrange for an interview with either the anesthesiologist or a nurse anesthetist who will go over your past medical history. You should be sure to disclose all of your medications at this time (including supplements, herbs, and over-the-counter drugs) so that the anesthesiologist can determine whether you need to stop taking them before surgery. Depending upon your health, the extent of the operation, and your hospital's policy, you could be admitted the night before the procedure. Many patients, however, come to the hospital the morning of the operation. You will be brought to the pre-op surgical suite, where you will change into a gown, and an intravenous catheter (an IV) will be inserted into your arm. You might be given a medication to help you relax. (Keep in mind that this is something you can ask for if you are feeling overly anxious.) You will then be placed on a moveable cot (or gurney) and wheeled into the operating room. At first glance, this might appear to be a cold, sterile place where everyone is wearing surgical gowns, masks, and hats. The surgical staff, however, will try to see that you are comfortable, and you will be able to talk to them. Once you are on the surgical table, the anesthesiologist will give you some medication into your vein to make you go to sleep. A tube will then be placed into your throat into which oxygen will be blown while you are asleep. You will sleep during the entire operation and wake up in the recovery room.

38. What does my surgeon mean when he or she says, "I got it all"? Does this mean I am cured?

When your surgeon says he or she got it all, what he is really saying is that they removed all the cancer they could see. Unfortunately, that does not necessarily mean a cure. We know that in many patients the cancer will come back—either at the original site or elsewhere in the body. Presumably, some cancer cells that were too small for the surgeon to see or for any scans to pick up must have escaped before the operation.

The pathologist will look to see whether the biopsy tumor from your surgery has **positive margins**. Positive margins mean that the cancer cells extend to the very edge of the biopsy or surgical sample. If so, there is a high likelihood that there were tumor cells remaining on the other side of the sample—the side remaining in the patient. Even if your resected tumor has **negative margins** (normal tissue at the edge of the biopsy sample), there is no way to determine if there were microscopic amounts of cancer cells left behind either in the area of the tumor or somewhere else in the body. Unfortunately, none of the blood tests, X-rays, or scans currently available is able to detect microscopic amounts of disease.

Many patients whose cancer recurs after surgery are confused and angry because they remember their surgeons saying they got it all. It is important to be aware that this does not mean there are no longer any cancer cells in your body, and you are cured. Although there is a considerable amount of research going on to detect smaller and smaller amounts of tumor, at this point the most accurate answer to the question, "Did the surgeon get it all?" is "We do not know."

Positive margins

A phrase used when cancer cells are found at the edge of the biopsy sample.

Negative margins

A phrase used when normal tissue is found at the edge of the biopsy sample.

Keep in mind that although successful lung surgery is reason to celebrate, you need to be vigilant about your follow-up care (see Question 91).

39. What should I expect following my surgery? What are the common complications of lung surgery?

When you wake up in the recovery room, you will be very woozy and might not realize where you are, or even that the operation is over. You will doze off and on while you are brought back to your room. If possible, it is often helpful to have a family member or loved one stay with you during those first few days. He or she can call the nurses for you, help make you comfortable, and assist you in getting around.

For the first 24 to 48 hours, you could be uncomfortable, but the nurses should respond to your request for pain medications. Ask your doctor if you can have **patient-controlled analgesia (PCA)**, a method by which you can regulate your own pain medication. By pressing a button attached to an IV, you can give yourself a small dose of morphine whenever you need it so that you do not have to wait for a nurse. The PCA machine is set so that you will not be able to overdose yourself.

You most likely will have a chest tube when you come out of surgery. This is a tube leading from the space between your lung and chest wall to a bag or container by your bedside. Suction is applied to drain the fluid and inflate the lung. Fortunately, this is not as painful or uncomfortable as it sounds! In addition, you will probably have a catheter leading from your bladder to a

Patient-controlled analgesia (PCA)

A method by which a patient can regulate the amount of pain medication he or she receives.

bag by the bedside (a Foley catheter). This is also pain-less and will drain your bladder until you are able to go to the bathroom by yourself. Most likely, you will also have oxygen prongs or a facemask for oxygen.

Despite the IVs and cath-eters, the nurse will get you up out of bed the first day following your surgery.

Despite the IVs and catheters, the nurse will get you up out of bed the first day following your surgery. This is very important to prevent post-op complications, such as blood clots and lung problems. A lung that is not breathing normally is very susceptible to accumulation of secretions, which in turn leads to accumulation of bacteria and pneumonia. In addition, the nurse or respi-ratory therapist will give you lung exercises to do to pre-vent this complication. It is important to have adequate pain control so that you feel like doing these exercises, so be sure to ask for and use pain medications as necessary.

You will not be allowed to eat or drink until the doc-tors are sure your stomach and intestines have woken up following the surgery. Typically, a patient's GI tract tends to stop working for several days following a gen-eral anesthesia. When you start passing gas from below, you will be allowed to drink clear liquids. Your diet will advance as your stomach and small intestine become more active.

The most common complication following lung surgery is infection—usually a lung infection, often from not breathing deeply and/or clearing secretions out of the lungs. Other unlikely complications are bleeding, infec-tions of the incision site, and post-operative heart prob-lems, such as congestive heart failure or an irregular heart rhythm.

Make sure that you have adequate pain medications to take home. It is not uncommon for surgeons to underestimate post-op pain. Patients are often sent home with a small supply of pain medication when, in reality, many will need to take some medications for a month or longer. If your doctor does not want to give you a large supply, make sure you know how to contact him or her for refills.

Healthy lifestyle behaviors post-surgery, including regular exercise, weight control and healthy nutrition have the potential to greatly reduce cancer-treatment associated morbidity and **mortality** in cancer survivors and can enhance quality of life. Recent research supports fitness as an important factor in long-tern survival, decreasing the likelihood of surgery complications as well as reducing fatigue in cancer survivors. In fact, you should ask your healthcare providers about including exercise as part of your post-surgery rehabilitation therapy.

Mortality
The number of people who die of a disease.

CHEMOTHERAPY

40. What is chemotherapy? How does it work?

Chemotherapy is a word for medications used to treat cancer. Unlike surgery and radiation, which are used to treat localized disease (in the lungs), chemotherapy is a systemic therapy used to treat disease that has spread to all parts of the body. Chemotherapy drugs are often administered intravenously (sometimes orally), and thus are absorbed into the blood. Since the blood flows to all parts of the body, in theory, cancer cells anywhere in the body would be exposed to the chemotherapy.

Chemotherapy works by interfering with the DNA of cancer cells (see Question 2). Because cancer cells divide rapidly and don't stop (uncontrolled growth), many chemotherapy drugs are specifically designed to target rapidly dividing cells. However, some normal cells in the body also grow rapidly—such as hair, the lining of the stomach, and blood cells—and chemotherapy can affect these cells as well, causing such side effects as hair loss, nausea (rarely vomiting), and susceptibility to infections. Ask your doctor about ways to prevent or reduce these side effects.

Regimen

Specific chemotherapy treatment plan involving the drugs, doses, and frequency of administration.

Chemotherapy sometimes consists of one drug, but more often it involves a combination of drugs called a **regimen**. Chemotherapy regimens combine drugs that have different mechanisms of action, or ways of attacking cancer cells, in order to increase their effectiveness and to prevent the cancer cells from developing resistance to chemotherapy. Your doctor will recommend possible chemotherapy regimens based on your type of lung cancer, your stage, the location of your disease, your general health, any previous treatments, the side effects of the drugs, and the goals of your treatment plan. For information on specific chemotherapy drugs and regimens used to treat lung cancer (see **Table 3**).

Above all, please note that the chemotherapy that is used to treat one type of cancer, such as breast cancer, colon cancer or prostate cancer, is very different from the chemotherapy used to treat lung cancer, and the side effects will be much different. Although support groups are very helpful in supporting you during your treatment, the side effects that some of the patients with other cancers have experienced are likely to be very different than the side effects experienced by lung cancer patients. In addition, there are many different chemotherapy regimens for lung cancers. These have different side effects, too. For example, some are more likely to cause hair loss than others. PLEASE talk to your doctor and/or nurse to get a realistic view of what YOU are likely to experience.

41. What can I expect during chemotherapy?

The typical chemotherapy session begins with a standard blood test called a **complete blood count (CBC)**. Because chemotherapy can lower your blood counts, your oncologist wants to be sure that your blood counts are high enough so that you are able to receive chemotherapy safely. (See Question 70 for a full explanation of how chemotherapy affects your blood.) You can ask your nurse or **phlebotomist** (a technician trained to draw blood) to use a small needle for your blood draw, which will minimize the discomfort caused when the needle is inserted into your vein.

The process of delivering IV chemotherapy is called an infusion. The most common IV method uses a thin needle or catheter (tiny plastic tube) that is inserted into a vein in your arm or hand. These IV needle sticks cause a bit more discomfort than a needle stick for a blood test because they require a slightly larger needle—the pain is a little sharper but just as fleeting. Some patients apply a numbing cream (Emla) prior to needle sticks to make the process virtually painless. You might want to ask your oncologist or oncology nurse if this might be an option for you.

Once inserted, the needle or catheter is taped down to prevent it from moving and causing any pain. The

Complete blood count (CBC)

A blood test that counts the number of white blood cells, red blood cells, and platelets.

Phlebotomist

A technician trained to draw blood.

The process of delivering IV chemotherapy is called an infusion. The most common IV method uses a thin needle or catheter (tiny plastic tube) that is inserted into a vein in your arm or hand.

chemotherapy drug(s)—and any pre-medications—are then dispensed from bags suspended from a metal IV pole. These liquids flow from the bags through a flexible tube that feeds into the needle or catheter in your vein. An infusion pump is sometimes used to deliver a precise amount of medication over a set period of time.

You will receive your pre-medications (pre-meds) first. These will likely include fluids for hydration and anti-emetics to prevent nausea and vomiting. Your oncology nurse should clearly explain the pre-meds and chemotherapy drugs you are getting. When the drugs begin to flow, you might feel a slight coldness or strange sensation at the IV site; however, the infusion process should be pain-free and uneventful. If you experience pain, burning, swelling, shortness of breath, or any other unusual reactions during your infusion, you should bring it to your nurse's attention immediately. Your nurse will check to see if the needle was inserted properly or perhaps adjust the flow of the medication to a more comfortable rate. There are other measures that can be taken to alleviate discomfort or other problems you might experience so you need to keep your nurse informed of your status.

The length of your infusion will depend on the number and amount of chemotherapy drugs you are receiving. Chemo sessions can take 1 hour, several hours, or several days. Extended infusions might require a hospital stay, although these are unusual for most lung cancer regimens. For the duration of your infusion, it often helps to watch TV, read a book, listen to music, talk to a friend, sleep—do whatever relaxes you and makes the time go more quickly. You are unlikely to experience any side effects during the infusion. When your infusion is over, be sure your nurse has told you about any potential side effects, what to do if you experience them, and under what circumstances you should call your doctor's office. If your nurse tells you that you could experience nausea, don't leave the office without a prescription for medications to prevent nausea, and be sure you know how to use them.

In some instances, chemotherapy can be administered outside an office or hospital setting. For example, oral chemotherapies—in pill, capsule, or liquid form—can be taken by patients at home. Portable infusion pumps allow some IV chemotherapies to be delivered at home as patients go about their usual activities.

42. What is a central line? What is a port? How do I know if I need one?

Patients typically receive chemotherapy intravenously through a thin needle that is inserted into a vein in the arm or hand. There are devices available called **central venous catheters** (**CVC**) that are semi-permanent IVs. They can remain in for extended periods of time (often months) and allow repeated access to larger veins without the pain or stress associated with IV needle sticks into the smaller, more delicate veins. CVCs require minor surgery for insertion but can be left in place indefinitely. There are two basic types of CVCs: external CVCs and ports (subcutaneous CVCs).

External CVCs. You might hear other patients talk about Broviac, Groshong, or Hickman catheters. These are names of common external CVCs. External CVCs are IVs which are inserted in a large blood vessel (usually the blood vessel underneath your clavicle, or collar bone), but the other end is exposed through the skin and

Central venous catheter (CVC)

A thin tube that is surgically inserted to allow access to large veins.

External CVCs

IVs inserted in a large blood vessel. The other end is exposed through the skin and capped off so a patient does not have to carry an IV bag with them all the time.

capped off so that one does not have to carry an IV bag around all the time. This allows for a convenient and pain-free IV for drawing blood and for delivering chemotherapy. They can also be used for blood transfusions, CT contrast, fluids, and nutrition. External CVCs require some care so that they won't become blocked by a blood clot or become infected. The risk of developing a blood clot can be reduced with the use of coumadin, a blood thinning medication. These types of lines are typically inserted by a surgeon as an outpatient procedure.

Pic-line

A type of central venous catheter inserted into a large vein in the arm.

Another type of external CVC is a **pic-line**, which is often inserted by a specialized nursing team. Unlike the external catheters described above, a pic-line is not inserted through the chest wall into the vein underneath the collar bone, or the subclavian vein. Instead, the pic-line is inserted into a large vein into the arm and then threaded up the arm into the subclavian vein. The advantages of pic-lines are that they can be put in relatively quickly by nurses; the disadvantage is that they usually do not stay in as long as some of the other external CVCs.

Port

A type of central venous catheter that is surgically implanted under the skin.

Ports. Another option for convenient venous access is a port—also known as a medi-port or port-a-cath (**Figure 2**). A port is a type of central venous catheter that is implanted wholly under the skin. Ports provide access to major veins but are not exposed through the skin as are external devices. They require much less care and carry less risk of infection than external CVCs. Although needle sticks must still be made through the skin, the discomfort is less than with an IV needle stick because a special needle is used, and the skin over the port toughens and becomes less sensitive over time. Numbing cream (Emla) can be applied to make this process completely pain-free. Unlike external CVCs, ports are minimally noticeable—they appear only as a small raised area under the skin. Ports require general anesthesia for insertion.

Neither external CVCs nor ports should significantly impact or change your daily activities. You can still bathe and exercise, for example, and neither is noticeable under clothing. Patients who should consider getting a venous access device include:

Neither external CVCs nor ports should significantly impact or change your daily activities.

- Patients who experience difficulty with blood drawing or chemotherapy IVs
- Patients who will be receiving chemotherapy on a frequent basis
- Patients who will be receiving chemotherapy drugs irritating to small veins

If you think you might benefit from having a venous access device such as an external CVC or a port, you should discuss this possibility with your oncologist. Most patients find that these devices greatly increase their quality of life during chemotherapy.

Skin
Subcutaneous tissue
Muscle

Figure 2 Schematic drawing of an implantable port.

Reprinted from Yarbro CH, Frogge MH, Goodman M, and Groenwald SL. *Cancer Nursing: Principles and Practice*, Sixth Edition. Sudbury, MA: Jones and Bartlett Publishers, LLC, 2005.

43. Why does my doctor order blood tests during my chemotherapy treatment?

Because chemotherapy attacks rapidly growing cells, it can affect your blood cells, which are among the most rapidly dividing cells in your body. This is one of the most common side effects of chemotherapy. Your blood contains white blood cells, red blood cells, and **platelets**, each of which has a specific function. If your chemotherapy treatment causes your blood counts (the number of your blood cells) to drop below normal, this can put you at risk for potentially dangerous side effects. In some cases, these effects can be prevented or controlled through the use of supportive therapies. Please note that some drugs cause more **myelosuppression** (drop in the blood counts) than others (see Table 3). Also, some drugs can affect one type of blood cell more than others. For example, while almost all drugs affect the white blood cells, Gemzar (gemcitabine) and carboplatin also lower the platelet count.

The drop in blood counts is usually temporary. The counts are often at their lowest between 10 to 14 days after the chemotherapy, at which point they start to bounce back. The counts are usually back to normal by the time the next treatment is to be delivered.

44. What can I expect from chemotherapy?

Although all chemotherapy has side effects, the reality is that most lung cancer patients tolerate chemotherapy relatively well. In fact, tales of nausea and vomiting—among the most feared effects of chemotherapy—date

Platelet

A type of blood cell responsible for clotting.

Myelosuppression

A decrease in the production of blood cells.

from years ago when chemotherapy drugs were more toxic and when effective anti-nausea drugs (**antiemetics**) were not available. Advances in medicine have led to the development of chemotherapy drugs with fewer and less severe side effects. In addition, oncologists can now provide patients with supportive therapies such as antiemetic drugs to prevent nausea and vomiting, medications to control pain, and growth factors to restore blood counts. It is important to remember that there is always something that can be done to eliminate, reduce, or help you cope with side effects from chemotherapy. The one possible exception is hair loss (**alopecia**). There are no effective ways to decrease hair loss by drugs that cause it, although not all chemotherapy drugs cause hair loss.

A comforting thought is that almost all chemotherapy side effects are temporary and resolve immediately following treatment. It helps to remind yourself of this whenever you are experiencing distressing effects. Infrequently, there can be side effects that persist after treatment and never go away completely. Patients who experience severe **peripheral neuropathy**, for example, often complain that they have residual tingling and numbness in their fingers and toes years after chemotherapy. There are also a small number of side effects that might appear after treatment is completed—so-called late effects. Although rare, these can be serious (for example, second cancers are considered late effects) and should be discussed with your oncologist prior to treatment. (See Question 78 for additional information on long-term and late effects.)

For additional information on side effects, see Part 7: Side Effects of Chemotherapy.

Antiemetics
Drugs that prevent nausea and vomiting.

Alopecia
Hair loss.

Peripheral neuropathy
Tingling, numbness, or burning sensation in hands, feet, or legs caused by damage to peripheral nerves by a tumor or by chemotherapy or radiation.

45. What is targeted therapy?

Unlike chemotherapy, which kills both normal (e.g., hair cells or blood cells) and cancer cells indiscriminately, many of these newer treatments are targeted at aspects of the cell that are specific for cancer—hence the term targeted therapies. Many of these drugs try to stop or inhibit chemical reactions, sometimes called pathways, which are active only in cancer cells and not normal cells. Interestingly, for many of these chemical reactions to occur, the pathway must *be activated* by a signal (or **ligand**) coming from outside the cell. This signal is usually a protein that does not diffuse into the cell. Instead, it binds to a molecule on the surface of the cell called a **receptor**. When this happens, the receptor becomes activated and starts the cascade or chain reaction of chemical reactions that eventually gets to the nucleus and activates abnormal, mutated genes. A theoretical advantage of these targeted therapies is that because they are specific for cancer cells and should not affect normal ones, the side effects associated with them should be much less. Indeed this is the case; these drugs rarely cause hair loss, nausea, or a drop in the blood counts.

Two major classes of drugs make up targeted therapies— antibodies and small molecules. The antibodies used for cancer are similar to the antibodies our bodies make to help fight infection. However, instead of attacking bacteria, these man-made antibodies attack the receptors on the outside surface of the cancer cell, and in doing so, block the initiation of the chemical cascade that causes the cells to grow and become cancerous. Antibodies are almost always given IV. Because our bodies will recognize them as foreign, they are sometimes associated with allergic (hypersensitivity) reactions.

Ligand

A molecule that binds to another chemical entity to form a larger complex.

Receptor

A protein molecule, embedded in either the plasma membrane or cytoplasm of a cell, to which a signaling molecule (or ligand) may attach.

Small molecules, on the other hand, are just what they sound like—molecules which are much smaller than antibodies and made to block specific pathways, or chemical reactions, on the inside of the cancer cell. Many of them are given in pill form. One class of small molecules you might hear about is called **tyrosine kinase inhibitors** or **TKIs**. TKIs block the activated part of the receptor on the inside of the cell and prevent it from starting the chain reaction.

In many cases, both antibodies and TKIs have been developed to target the same pathway. In some instances, it is not known which is better—the antibody or the small molecule.

A number of different areas of investigation can be lumped under the term targeted therapies. Two general categories approved for the treatment for lung cancer include:

- **Growth factor inhibitors**. As mentioned in Question 2, cancer cells are often stimulated to grow by substances called growth factors. Two are of particular interest in lung cancer.

- The **epidermal growth factor** (**EGF**) is a protein or ligand made by some cancer cells and is secreted into the space surrounding the cancer cell and the rest of the cancer cells that make up the tumor. EGF doesn't directly diffuse into a cancer cell; instead, it binds to its receptor on the outside of the cell. Binding of the EGF to the EGF receptor (**EGFR**) activates the receptor, causing a chemical chain reaction that eventually ends up in the nucleus of the cell, stimulating the cell to grow.

Tyrosine kinase inhibitors (TKIs)

Small molecules which block the activated part of the receptor on the inside of the cancer cell and prevent it from starting a chemical reaction which causes the cell to grow and divide.

Growth factor inhibitors

Substances that inhibit the growth factors that stimulate cells to grow.

Epidermal growth factor (EGF)

A protein made by cancer cells that causes cancer cells around them to grow and divide.

EGFR

The receptor on the surface of the cancer cell to which EGF binds.

A number of different drugs are being developed to stop EGF from activating the receptor and/or stopping the chain reaction that tells the DNA to start to grow and divide. Some of these drugs work by blocking the EGF from attaching to its receptor (these are usually antibodies to the receptor and come in IV form; cetuximab or Erbitux is an example); others (TKIs) work by preventing the activated receptor from sending chemical signals to the nucleus. Tarceva (erlotinib) is an example of this latter kind of drug, which usually comes in oral form. At this point, it is not known whether either approach is better than the other. However, Tarceva is rarely given at the same time as chemotherapy (concurrently), whereas Erbitux is rarely given alone. Of the two, currently only Tarceva is approved in the United States for lung cancer.

It is not clear which patients benefit from one of the EGFR inhibitors. Obviously, if your tumor doesn't have any EGFR, you do not have the target for these targeted drugs, and it would seem unlikely you would benefit. However, nearly everyone with lung cancer (85%–90%) has at least some EGFR on the surface of their cancer cells. Since not everyone benefits, scientists are studying the tumors to see if they can predict who is most likely to respond.

In some patients, the EGFR on their tumor is not only over-expressed (the cancer cell has too much of it) but is also mutated. Patients who have a mutation in their EGFR are more likely to have a response (e.g., shrinkage of disease) than those patients whose tumors over-express EGFR, although these patients too can benefit. However, only about 10% of North Americans and Europeans are likely to have a mutation. Nevertheless, both groups of patients (those whose tumors have a lot of receptor [over-expression] and those whose tumors have a mutated EGFR) could benefit by shrinkage of their disease, delayed growth, and improved survival. However, the benefit is more likely in the patients with EGFR mutated tumors.

Although some patients can have a long-lasting dramatic response to Tarceva, in most patients the tumor starts to grow again at some point. Scientists have identified several reasons for this, including the fact that some of these cells can develop a new mutation which stops Tarceva from binding to the receptor (called a T790M resistance mutation). There are many clinical trials going on to identify ways to overcome this resistance mutation, as well as other mechanisms of resistance that have been identified.

Tomma adds...

"We have now discovered that I have the EGFR mutation which is associated with lung cancer. So I have learned that being an informed lung cancer patient is much more important than worrying about what might have caused it!"

- **EML-4/ALK fusion protein** (also known as ALK positive) is another example of a chemical reaction in the cell gone wrong. In this case, two genes, which were located on two different chromosomes, break apart from their usual chromosome and join together. (The assay used to identify this abnormality is called a break apart assay.) The resultant protein also starts a cascade of chemical reactions ultimately ending up in the nucleus of the cell, causing the cell to grow. A drug called Xalkori (crizotinib) is very good at

EML-4/ALK fusion protein

An abnormal protein made when two genes combine (e.g., the EML-4 gene and the ALK gene). The resulting protein can cause cancer cells to grow and divide.

inhibiting this, and very dramatic responses have been seen in patients who have this EML-4/ALK fusion protein. This drug was recently approved by the FDA for these patients and represents a remarkable development of a targeted drug—from identification of the EML-4/ALK fusion protein to identification of a drug that targeted that protein to clinical trials to FDA approval was a mere 4 years. Although this might not sound quick, consider that it took about 10 years for Tarceva to be approved.

As with EGFR mutations, the EML-4/ALK fusion protein is most commonly found in patients who have never smoked—about 20% of them will have this molecular aberration. Generally, patients who have an EGFR mutation do not have the EML-4/ALK fusion protein, and those who have the EML-4/ALK fusion protein do not have an EGFR mutation. They are mutually exclusive. Xalkori is generally very well tolerated but has one unusual side effect. Some people have described an unusual blurriness of their vision when turning their head rapidly. This does not appear to have any serious consequences and goes away once the drug has been stopped. As with Tarceva, the cancer starts to grow again in some patients, and scientists are trying to identify how the cell becomes resistant to Xalkori.

Angiogenesis inhibitors

Drugs that prevent the formation of new blood vessels.

- **Angiogenesis inhibitors.** As discussed in Question 2, tumors need a constant and growing blood supply to feed them, much like an advancing army needs a constant and growing supply of food and materials to sustain it. Blocking off this blood supply should, in theory, have two effects. It should choke off the cancer by stopping the flow of oxygen and nutrients to it, and it should stop the tumor from spreading through its usual highway—the bloodstream. Avastin, or bevacizumab, is the first of these agents approved for lung cancer. Avastin is an antibody, similar to the antibodies that block the EGF pathway mentioned above. However, Avastin blocks a growth signal called **VEGF (vascular endothelial growth factor)** from binding to its receptor on the surface of blood vessel cells, not cancer cells. VEGF stimulates the blood vessel cells (endothelial cells) to grow, divide, and migrate into the tumor. As with the EGF pathway, a number of small molecules or TKIs are being developed to prevent the activated receptor from sending chemical signals to the nucleus. This is a promising area of cancer research with many new and ongoing clinical trials in lung cancer.

VEGF (vascular endothelial growth factor)

A family of growth factors, most often made by tumors, that causes blood vessel cells (vascular cells) to grow into the tumor.

46. What are common side effects of targeted therapies?

Major side effects of EGFR inhibitors, such as Tarceva (erlotinib) or Erbitux (cetuximab), include rash and, less commonly, diarrhea. The rash looks like acne and is typically scattered over the trunk and face. In some patients, it can be severe. If you develop a severe rash, talk to your doctor. He or she will probably prescribe skin creams or antibiotics and might reduce your dose.

A common side effect of angiogenesis inhibitors is hypertension. Your doctor should be monitoring you for high blood pressure and, if need be, giving you blood pressure medications or adding to or changing the ones you are currently on. Another somewhat less common side effect is the loss of very small amounts of protein in the urine. Your physician could ask you to give periodic urine samples to check for this. A rare side effect of these drugs is coughing up blood, particularly in patients with squamous cell carcinoma. If this happens to you, notify your doctor at once because, very rarely, some patients with squamous cell carcinoma have died of this complication. Because of this, Avastin is limited to patients without squamous cell carcinoma and those with no history of coughing up blood. Some doctors will also withhold Avastin or other angiogenic inhibitors from patients with large tumors that are located next to large blood vessels, although this has not been definitely shown to be a risk factor for bleeding.

RADIATION THERAPY

47. What is radiation therapy, and how does it work?

Radiation therapy (also sometimes referred to as radiotherapy, X-ray therapy, or irradiation) is the use of high-energy rays to stop cancer cells from growing or multiplying.

Radiation treatment is carefully planned to deliver as much radiation as possible to tumor cells while doing as little damage as possible to normal surrounding cells.

Radiation causes damage to the DNA, which is often permanent, causing cells to die. After cell death, the cellular remains must eventually disintegrate and be removed from the body. This dead cell removal can be quite slow and there could be a delay in the shrinkage of tumors receiving radiation even though all the cells are dead. It affects normal and abnormal cells in the area being treated.

Radiation treatment is carefully planned to deliver as much radiation as possible to tumor cells while doing as little damage as possible to normal surrounding cells. Radiation is usually given in small doses over a long period of time to increase the effect on the tumor cells while providing intervals between treatments to allow injured normal tissues to recover, thus reducing the side effects of radiation.

48. What is a dose of radiation? How many treatments will I need?

The dose of radiation is measured in units called **rads** or **Gray (Gy)**. One hundred rads equals one Gy or 100 **centigray**. The typical dose of radiation is about 6,000 rads or 6,000 centigray or 60 Gy. Rather than administer all 60 Gy in one treatment, the radiation is divided up into many treatments. The total dose of radiation and the number of treatments you will need depends on the size, location, and type of your cancer.

Rad
Unit of radiation.

Gray (Gy)
Modern unit of radiation dosage. 100 rads is equal to one Gy.

Centigray
Unit of radiation; same as a rad.

Radiation delivered with curative intent usually consists of about 60 Gy given two Gy at a time, in 30 treatments or **fractions**, although your doctor will determine the best dose and number of fractions best for you. Treatments are typically given daily, although occasionally specific reasons require that treatment be given more frequently (twice a day) or less frequently (two to three times a week). Usually, radiation is given 5 days a week, Monday through Friday, over 6 weeks. Some data suggest that, in certain situations, giving the radiation therapy twice per day for a total of 12 days might be more effective than the standard schedule.

Fraction
Single treatment of radiation. The total dose of radiation is usually given over multiple fractions.

Radiation oncologists are also developing ways to give even higher doses of radiation (70 Gy or more) without damaging surrounding tissue. When delivered to the brain, for example, it is sometimes given by a device called the gamma knife, cyber knife (depending upon

Stereotactic Body Radiation Therapy (SBRT)

A way of delivering very high doses of radiation to the tumor in 3–5 fractions, without damaging surrounding normal tissues.

the type of device), or radiosurgery. When delivered elsewhere in the body, it is sometimes called **Stereotactic Body Radiation Therapy**, or **SBRT**.

The amount of radiation given to reduce symptoms (palliative radiation) is usually less than what is given in an attempt to cure the patient. This is because smaller doses of radiation can shrink the tumor enough to reduce symptoms and have fewer side effects than high-dose radiation.

49. What equipment is used to deliver radiation?

A variety of specialized equipment is used in both planning and treatment with radiation therapy. An X-ray machine called a simulator is used during the planning phase. A computer might also be used. The simulator and computer help determine the best plan for the area that needs to be treated (**treatment fields**).

Treatment field

The area of the body that is radiated.

The treatment is usually delivered with a type of equipment called a linear accelerator that produces high-energy X-rays. Modern advances in the linear accelerator, or **linac,** have made it the most commonly used equipment. Cobalt accelerators are an older technology that is much less commonly used and produces a different type of energy beam called gamma rays.

Linac

A linear accelerator that produces high-energy X-rays for radiation therapy.

50. What can I expect during radiation therapy? What is the actual procedure like, and how long does each treatment take?

Your first visit to the radiation therapy department lasts 1 to 3 hours and usually does not include any treatments. A radiation oncologist will review your records and examine you to decide whether radiation therapy is appropriate and which treatment plan is best. He or she will discuss treatment recommendations with you, including how many treatments are needed and what their effects are likely to be. This is the time to ask questions. Your next appointment will be for a treatment planning CT or a **simulation**, and you might not see the doctor.

The purpose of the simulation visit is to plan the technical aspects of your treatments. A therapist will take you to the simulator room where he or she will accurately plan your radiation treatments. Simulators are not treatment machines; they are specialized machines built to mimic X-ray treatment units and to take moving or still X-ray pictures. During your simulation, X-rays might be taken. In some cases a computerized tomography (CT) simulator is used to further refine treatment planning.

A variety of methods is used to line up your treatment field correctly. A special mold could be made for you to lie in during your treatment. Tiny dots might be tattooed on your skin to mark the center and corners of your field. These look like tiny freckles and will not be visible to anyone except those who know where to look. Oil-based markers or ink could also be used to mark your skin. It is important that you do not wash the marks off until all the treatments are completed. These marks stay on best if they are not allowed to get wet for

Simulation

Planning the radiation fields with a CT scan.

the first 24 hours; after that, you can bathe or shower. The water can run over the marks, but you should not use soap or a washcloth on the marked area. When the marks fade, the therapist touches them up at the treatment unit. The markings will rub off on clothes, so it's recommended that you wear older clothing. Pretreating the garment with a stain remover or hair spray before washing will generally remove the stain. This simulation planning session usually takes 1 to 2 hours. You might get a treatment on this day, depending on whether special blocks need to be made for your treatment and whether there is an opening in the treatment schedule.

Most patients are treated on an outpatient basis. If you live too far away from the radiation center to commute from home, you might consider staying with local friends or relatives or in a nearby motel. Many hospitals have arrangements with nearby motels for a lower cost for their radiation patients. The treatment schedule can generally be tailored to accommodate at least a part-time work schedule.

Radiotherapy treatments are very similar to having X-rays.

Radiotherapy treatments are very similar to having X-rays. Just as you are not able to see, feel, or hear the rays in a chest X-ray, there is no pain or discomfort with the actual radiation treatment. If you are in pain for other reasons, the treatment process could be uncomfortable because you will be required to lie still for a short period of time. Patients experiencing pain are encouraged to take pain medications 1 hour before a radiotherapy visit.

It is absolutely essential to remain in exactly the same position during the treatment so the radiation beam is always reaching the exact treatment area, rather than any surrounding tissue. Therapists use molds and other devices to minimize movement and to duplicate the identical position for each treatment.

A therapist will position you under the appropriate machine and then leave the room for the few minutes the machine is on. Because therapists work with radiation every day, it is essential that they leave the room during treatments to avoid getting too much exposure to radiation. The therapist does, however, stay nearby to monitor via television and can communicate with you through a microphone in the treatment room.

Treatments usually take about 10 minutes each day. The machine is on for only about 1 minute for each treatment field; most people have at least two fields. Patients can also expect some waiting time before their actual treatment. The treatment time could be longer if: 1) patients are treated on two different machines or have many fields or 2) patients have a large field or a complicated set-up.

51. Are there advances in radiation therapy that I should know about?

Advances in radiation technology are allowing more effective treatment of tumors while decreasing the incidence of side effects. **Three-dimensional conformal radiation therapy** (**3D-CRT**) is a technology that enables doctors to deliver higher doses of radiation to the lung tumor more precisely by using a CT scanner to provide a more accurate measurement of the tumor and its location. Thus, effective doses of radiation can be administered to tumors with less damage to normal tissue. A new type of 3D-CRT technology called **intensity modulated radiation therapy** (**IMRT**) is currently

Advances in radiation technology are allowing more effective treatment of tumors while decreasing the incidence of side effects.

Three-dimensional conformal radiation therapy (3D-CRT)

A type of radiation therapy that enables higher doses of radiation to be delivered more precisely than standard radiation therapy.

Intensity Modulated Radiation Therapy (IMRT)

A type of three-dimensional radiation therapy (3D-CRT) that uses radiation beams of varying strengths.

under investigation. IMRT promises to further increase the effectiveness of radiation treatment by using radiation beams of varying strengths. Tumors are irregular in thickness and shape, and IMRT technology can control the intensity of radiation delivered to different parts of the tumor, thereby increasing tumor kill and decreasing radiation-induced side effects. Stereotactic body radiotherapy (SBRT) is another high-precision technology under investigation for treatment of lung tumors.

Your radiation oncologist can tell you whether any of these technologies might be appropriate treatment options for you.

52. What are the common side effects of radiation therapy?

To get to the tumor, the beam of radiation has to pass through all the tissues in front of and behind the tumor, thereby generating side effects in these normal tissues. For example, radiation to a tumor in the chest must pass in through the skin, the normal lung, the tumor, and then go out through normal lung behind the tumor and the skin. If the tumor is near the esophagus (or feeding tube) or spinal cord it might pass through a portion of these as well. Because of these side effects, radiation cannot be administered to the entire body; instead, it must be limited to the areas of tumor. The amount of radiation that any one area of the body can tolerate varies. Normal tissues that are extremely sensitive to the effects of radiation, and thus don't tolerate it well, include organs within the abdomen and the spinal cord.

The side effects of radiation relate to the amount and nature of normal tissues through which the beam of radiation must pass, as well as to the total dose of radiation given. Therefore, side effects will vary from patient to patient depending upon each patient's treatment plan. In general, however, common side effects of high-dose (60 Gy, or 6000 rads) radiation on various body tissues are as follows:

- *Skin.* Radiation side effects to the skin can include a sunburn-like rash. For lung cancer patients, this is rarely a major problem.

- *Normal lungs.* Radiation can cause irritation of the lungs (**pneumonitis**), which can result in shortness of breath and cough. In some patients, this can result in permanent scarring of the lungs (**fibrosis**). Although these side effects are mild and well tolerated in most patients, in some patients with underlying poor lung function, the loss of breath is so significant that the patient could end up on oxygen permanently. Sometimes, the radiation oncologist will prescribe steroids if he or she thinks radiation pneumonitis or fibrosis is the cause of the breathing problem.

- *Esophagus.* The esophagus is the tube through which food travels from the mouth to the stomach. Because it passes through the very center of the chest, it often gets exposed to radiation and can become irritated. Irritation of the esophagus usually feels like a sore throat, which can sometimes be so bad that patients have a hard time swallowing solid foods. This is a temporary side effect that usually occurs 3 to 4 weeks into the radiation treatment and continues for about 2 weeks afterward. Rarely, this irritation can cause scarring or fibrosis of the esophagus, which can result in problems with food getting stuck. If this happens, the patient might need an upper endoscopy, in which a gastroenterologist looks

Pneumonitis
Irritation of the lungs.

Fibrosis
Scarring.

down into the esophagus with a fiber-optic tube or an endoscope and then uses a balloon at the end of the endoscope to squeeze open the scar tissue and dilate the esophagus.

If the sore throat experienced during radiation therapy becomes too bad, many radiation therapists prescribe a liquid medication containing some lidocaine. Lidocaine can numb the throat, making it easier to eat. During this period of time, do not worry about eating a balanced meal, meat, or solids. It is more important to stay hydrated and consume as many calories as you can, usually in the form of high-protein or calorie shakes, puddings, creamed soups, and the like.

Recent studies in NSCLC patients undergoing chemoradiation treatment found that the drug amifostine (Ethyol) might reduce treatment-related esophageal symptoms. Ask your doctor if a **radioprotectant**, such as amifostine, is available to you.

Radioprotectant

A medication that reduces certain side effects of radiation.

- *Heart.* It is rare to experience heart problems from radiation. The radiotherapist is usually able to direct the beam of radiation so that only small areas of the heart are exposed.

- *Spine.* The spinal cord is very sensitive to radiation and therefore cannot tolerate high doses. Indeed, this is often a factor that limits the amount of radiation that can be delivered because side effects from spinal radiation are usually permanent. Irritation of the spinal cord can cause back pain and, rarely, numbness, tingling, and weakness of one of the legs, which, in extremely rare cases, can lead to paralysis.

- *Fatigue.* Fatigue is one of the most common side effects of radiation therapy. It is important that you get enough rest during this period. While fatigue can last from 6 weeks to 12 months after your last radiation treatment, it usually gets better 1 to 2 weeks after the treatment is finished.

COMBINED MODALITY THERAPY

53. What is combined modality therapy for lung cancer? What are the advantages and disadvantages of this approach?

Combined modality therapy usually means receiving two or more types of treatment: a local treatment (such as radiotherapy or surgery) and systemic chemotherapy. This is usually recommended when a patient has Stage II or locally advanced (Stage III) disease. Combined modality therapy is recommended because such patients often have a high chance of recurrence—either locally (at the site of the original tumor) or distantly (somewhere else in the body). In the latter case, if the cancer comes back somewhere else in the body, it is not the fault of the surgeon—presumably some cancer cells must have spread (metastasized) before the operation. A local recurrence also does not mean that the surgeon did not do his or her job—it means that microscopic amounts of cancer cells, too small for the surgeon to see, were left behind. Therefore, two types of treatment are needed: therapy aimed at the tumor itself (surgery or radiation) and therapy aimed at cancer cells that might have already escaped (chemotherapy or targeted therapy).

The subject of combined modality treatment, and how to administer it, is one of the biggest areas of controversy among lung oncologists. When should the doctor give the chemo? Before radiation or surgery? After? Which

The subject of combined modality treatment, and how to administer it, is one of the biggest areas of controversy among lung oncologists.

type of local treatment should you have—radiation or surgery? Both? Should the chemotherapy be given at the same time as the radiation? Which chemotherapy is best? Because medical knowledge regarding combination therapy is evolving, you should discuss the pros and cons of each of these approaches with your doctor.

One of the potential disadvantages of combined modality therapy is enhanced side effects.

- If high-dose radiation (60 Gy, or 6000 rads) is given before surgery, the normal tissues become so affected that the body has a hard time healing, and patients can have problems with wounds breaking apart inside the chest. Lower doses of radiation (45 Gy, or 4500 rads) are better tolerated preoperatively.

- Chemotherapy given concurrently (at the same time) with radiation instead of sequentially (one after the other), in particular, can have more side effects. Patients tend to experience many more problems with fatigue, sore throat, and swallowing. In addition, they are more likely to suffer from radiation pneumonitis and fibrosis (see Question 53). Nevertheless, because there is a survival advantage when the treatment is given this way, it is often recommended, particularly for patients with good performance status (see Question 34).

How Will My Doctor Decide Which Treatment is Best for Me?

What are the standard treatment options for my stage of NSCLC?

What is personalized medicine?

What are the standard treatment options for my stage of SCLC?

More . . .

TREATMENT OF NSCLC

54. What are the standard treatment options for my stage of NSCLC?

The standard treatment of NSCLC depends upon several factors, including the stage of the disease and the patient's general health. The first of these will determine which treatment will be recommended; the second will determine whether the treatment needs to be changed in some way.

Please note that the following treatment recommendations are generalizations only. You must talk to your oncologist about your specific case. He or she might change these recommendations based upon the specific circumstances of your situation or your underlying health. In addition, advances in the treatment of lung cancer are being made every day; what is recommended today (or in this book) will almost certainly be outdated tomorrow. An excellent source for current information on lung cancer treatment is the NCI/PDQ Treatment Summaries, which can be found on the National Cancer Institute's website, *www.cancer.gov*, or the website of the American Society of Clinical Oncology, *www.cancer.net*.

Stages I & II NSCLC

Stage I NSCLC is a tumor that is usually relatively small (less than 3 centimeters, or 1½ inches) and does not involve any lymph nodes. The standard therapy for Stage I NSCLC is surgery, preferably a lobectomy if the patient's underlying lung function is okay and a wedge resection if it is not. With surgery, the chances of being cured of this cancer run between 60%–80%. Some patients, however, cannot tolerate even a wedge resection because their lung function is so poor; other patients could have such significant heart disease that they cannot tolerate any operation. In these cases, high-dose radiation can sometimes be given, although it is less likely to be curative compared to surgery.

The most common examples of Stage II NSCLC are a tumor that has spread to the local lymph nodes (also called hilar nodes, or **N1 nodes**); OR a tumor that is growing into the chest wall but does not have any lymph node involvement; OR a particularly large tumor. In these cases, surgery is recommended.

N1 nodes

Hilar nodes (e.g., nodes at the base of the lung).

Despite the fact that the tumor has been successfully removed, there is a chance it could come back, either in the lung or elsewhere (see Question 69). **Adjuvant chemotherapy** is chemotherapy given after surgery, and it has been shown to reduce the chance of lung cancer coming back after lung surgery for patients with Stage II disease and some patients with Stage I disease who have very large tumors. This is a relatively new finding and some doctors might not be aware of it. So if you have had surgery for Stage I or Stage II lung cancer, be sure to ask your doctor whether you might need adjuvant chemotherapy.

Adjuvant chemotherapy

Therapy given after surgery in case any cancer cells have been left behind.

Areas of Research and Clinical Trials (see also Questions 59 and 60)

Although most patients with Stage I lung cancer are cured of their disease, some are not. Lung cancer doctors are exploring several major areas of research for early stage (Stage I and II) patients:

- Can a **chemopreventive agent** prevent the development of lung cancer? In addition to their risk of recurrent disease, patients who develop one lung cancer are at higher risk of developing a second. This

Chemopreventive agent

A natural or synthetic substance used to prevent cancer.

risk exists primarily for smokers or former smokers because the carcinogens in tobacco smoke are inhaled into both lungs and could have caused mutations in more than one place. **Chemoprevention** refers to the use of a substance, such as a drug or vitamin, to prevent cancer. There are several large clinical trials looking at the possible role of certain drugs as chemopreventive agents.

- Is **neoadjuvant chemotherapy** helpful? Neoadjuvant chemotherapy is a term for chemotherapy that is given before surgery to kill any microscopic cancer cells that could have already spread, or metastasized, elsewhere in the body. It is given prior to surgery because patients are likely to be stronger and better able to tolerate it and to attack the microscopic metastases while they are still small.

- What is the role of **radiofrequency ablation (RFA)**? RFA uses high-frequency electric current to kill cancer cells, and some people feel that it can be used instead of surgery. However, this has never been proven; we do not know how it compares to surgery.

- Radiation. Stereotactic body radiotherapy (SBRT) and three-dimensional conformal radiation therapy (3D-CRT), including intensity modulated radiation therapy (IMRT), are all different methods of administering high doses of radiation that are more precise than traditional radiotherapy (see Question 47). Research is underway to determine if administering higher doses with fewer side effects will increase the effectiveness of these radiation techniques in the treatment of lung tumors.

Stage III NSCLC

Stage III NSCLC is a cancer that is big, bulky, and difficult or impossible to resect but has no obvious signs of

Chemoprevention

The use of natural or synthetic substances to prevent cancer.

Neoadjuvant chemotherapy

Therapy given before the primary therapy; for example, neoadjuvant chemotherapy, which is sometimes given prior to surgery.

Radiofrequency ablation (RFA)

Treatment that uses high-frequency electric current to kill cancer cells.

metastatic spread. It is typically subdivided into two sub-stages: Stage IIIA, which usually refers to a tumor that is technically operable from a surgeon's viewpoint, and Stage IIIB, which is not operable. Because the cancer is so large, and has spread to mediastinal lymph nodes, the chance that it has already escaped and gone into the blood stream or lymphatics is high. Thus, whether or not to undergo surgery for Stage IIIA is somewhat controversial; many doctors feel high doses of radiation treatment, not surgery, are the best local treatment. Regardless, the chances that the cancer has spread are so high that chemotherapy is almost always used as well.

Stage IIIA

Common examples of Stage IIIA disease include:

- Mediastinal lymph node involvement (N2 disease)
- A tumor that is growing into the chest wall and has lymph node involvement (either hilar or mediastinal)

Stage IIIA disease is one disease stage for which combined modality therapy has definitely been shown to improve survival over single-agent therapy alone. Again, clinical trials are ongoing to determine which of the following options is best:

- Preoperative (neoadjuvant) chemotherapy followed by surgery
- Preoperative chemotherapy and radiation therapy followed by surgery
- Surgery followed by post-operative (adjuvant) chemotherapy
- Chemotherapy followed by radiation or radiation followed by chemotherapy
- Chemotherapy given at the same time (concurrently) as radiation therapy

Stage IIIA disease is one disease stage for which combined modality therapy has definitely been shown to improve survival over single-agent therapy alone.

Stage IIIB

Common examples of Stage IIIB disease:

- A tumor that is growing into the heart, trachea, or one of the large vessels leading into or out of the heart
- A tumor with mediastinal lymph nodes on the opposite side of the tumor (e.g., a left-sided tumor with right-sided mediastinal lymph nodes)
- Patients whose tumor has spread to a different lobe in the same lung (e.g., a right lower lung tumor with a metastases to the right lower lobe). This is called **T4** disease.

T4

A tumor that invades the mediastinum, heart, ribs or spine, or any of the major structures in the chest OR has spread to another area in the same lobe.

In all of these cases, the surgeon cannot completely resect the entire tumor. If all of the tumor cannot be completely resected, surgery is generally NOT recommended. Surgery can be painful, can have side effects or complications, and is rarely curative in this situation. Therefore, it is generally thought that it is not helpful to operate on a patient's tumor unless you can get it all. In addition, incision lines that contain a few microscopic leftover tumor cells have a very hard time healing so these patients are at increased risk for post-operative complications.

Treatment of Stage IIIB disease usually involves chemotherapy and radiation therapy, although the use of radiation therapy in patients with T4 disease is somewhat controversial, as it is difficult to give radiation to such large areas of the lung.

Most studies show that it is more effective to give the chemotherapy and radiation therapy at the same time (concurrent chemo/rads) rather than one after the other (sequentially), even though it has side effects.

Areas of Research and Clinical Trials (see also Questions 59–60)

The treatment of Stage IIIB disease is a very active area of research. Questions that are being explored include:

- Should patients receive additional chemotherapy either before or after the concurrent chemo/rads?

- If the chemo is given at the same time as the radiation, should it be given in standard doses (e.g., high doses every 3 weeks) or weekly, at lower doses? Should both high-dose chemotherapy and weekly low-dose chemo with radiotherapy be given, and, if so, in what order? What are the best chemotherapy drugs for this situation?

- For those patients who have completed their chemo-radiotherapy, and in whom the tumor appears to have stopped growing, is there anything else that can be given afterward to prevent it from growing?

Stage IV NSCLC

Roughly half of all lung cancer patients will be diagnosed with Stage IV disease—metastatic disease, or disease involving a pleural effusion. Unfortunately, at this time, the prospects for cure from Stage IV lung cancer are not good. Therefore, the goals of treatment are to prevent the cancer from growing for as long as possible and reduce symptoms and, in doing so, improve both quality of life and survival. Because the cancer has spread, a local therapy is usually not recommended, unless it is to reduce specific symptoms, such as radiotherapy given to help with a painful bony metastasis.

Generally speaking, chemotherapy for patients with Stage IV NSCLC usually involves a combination of two drugs (a **doublet**). In the past, one of the two drugs has been a platin, such as cisplatin or carboplatin (commonly

Doublet chemotherapy

Two chemotherapy drugs used together.

Platin doublet

One of the two drugs in the doublet is either cisplatin or carboplatin.

Schedule

How frequently chemotherapy is given.

Cycle

The schedule of administration of chemotherapy that is repeated four–six times.

Typically, patients receive two to three cycles of chemotherapy and then have a CT scan to determine if the chemotherapy is working.

Stable

Cancer has stopped growing following treatment.

Responding

Cancer that has shrunk in response to chemotherapy.

called a **platin doublet**), although this does not necessarily have to be the case. The different two-drug regimens differ in how frequently they are given (the **schedule**), how much they cost, and their side effects. In the past, most regimens were about the same in terms of effectiveness; however, it might be that some of the newer drugs will be more effective.

Chemotherapy regimens are given on a regular schedule called a **cycle**. Most (but not all) cycles are every 3 weeks. For example, a typical 3-week cycle involves giving the drug on *day 1* and then coming back on *day 21* for the next cycle. Some drugs might be given more than once during a cycle. Gemcitabine, for example, is given on days 1 and 8 of a 21-day cycle. The vast majority of regimens are given as an outpatient.

Typically, patients receive two to three cycles of chemotherapy and then have a CT scan to determine if the chemotherapy is working. Remember—doctors are happy if the tumor is the same size or smaller, as long as it is not bigger. If the cancer is **stable** (e.g., the same size) or **responding** (smaller), the doctor will give another two–three cycles and again repeat the scan. The doctor usually stops after four–six cycles because most studies have shown that more is not helpful, and the side effects, particularly fatigue and myelosuppression, tend to catch up with a person.

Avastin (bevacizumab) is often given in combination with chemotherapy to patients who do not have squamous cell carcinoma and are not at risk for other complications (ask your doctor). There is some data to suggest that Erbitux (cetuximab) could also be helpful, although at the time of this writing, it has not yet been approved for NSCLC.

A number of different chemotherapy regimens are used for the treatment of advanced NSCLC (see **Table 3**). The regimens differ in terms of their side effects, cost, and how frequently they are given. It is beyond the scope of this book to discuss the pros and cons of each. Indeed, by the time this book is published, almost certainly more will have been approved. You should have a frank discussion with your medical oncologist regarding the pros and cons of the different regimens.

A relatively new concept that has arisen is **maintenance therapy**. Maintenance therapy involves a single drug that is given at the completion of the four to six cycles of the doublet chemotherapy to those patients whose disease has not grown during the chemotherapy. It is supposed to maintain the response to the doublet chemotherapy. At the time of this writing, three drugs have been approved for maintenance therapy: Avastin, Tarceva, and Alimta.

Maintenance therapy

A single drug given indefinitely after standard doublet chemotherapy to maintain the remission.

An active area of research is around the appropriate role of maintenance therapy. Should everyone get it? What is the best maintenance therapy? Continuing one of the drugs in the original doublet (continuation maintenance) or switching to something new (switch maintenance)?

55. What is genomics?

Genomics is a term for the study of the abnormal genes that cause a person's particular cancer. As discussed in Question 2, mutated genes are a common cause of cancer. In some cases, a particular mutation will cause a specific type of cancer. For example, a mutated EGFR gene causes adenocarcinoma of the lung (see Questions 2 and 45). This is sometimes called a **driver mutation**, meaning

Driver mutation

A mutation which causes a cancer cell to grow and divide; without this specific mutation, the cancer cell would die.

Table 3 Selected side effects of drugs which are commonly used for the treatment of lung cancer*

Drugs which cause myelo-suppression (a temporary drop in the blood counts): • Taxol (paclitaxel) • Taxotere (docetaxel) • Cytoxan (cyclophosphamide) • Adriamycin (doxorubicin) • Vespid (etoposide) • Navelbine (vinorelbine) • Carboplatin • Topotecan • Gemzar (gemcitabine)	Drugs which usually cause minimal or no myelosuppression: • Cisplatin • Alimta (pemetrexed) • Avastin (bevacizumab) • Tarceva (erlotinib) • Erbitux (cetuximab) • Xalkori (crizotinib)	
Drugs which are likely to cause almost complete hair loss: • Taxol (paclitaxel) • Taxotere (docetaxel) • Cytoxan (cyclophosphamide) • Adriamycin (doxorubicin)	Drugs which cause mild to moderate hair loss: • Vespid (etoposide) • Navelbine (vinorelbine) • Carboplatin • Topotecan • Gemzar (gemcitabine)	Drugs which usually cause only mild or no hair loss: • Cisplatin • Alimta (pemetrexed)
Drugs which will cause nausea, unless the proper anti-emetics are given: • Cisplatin	Drugs which can cause mild nausea (usually well controlled by anti-emetics): • Taxol (paclitaxel) • Taxotere (docetaxel) • Carboplatin • Gemzar (gemcitabine) • Navelbine (vinorelbine) • Topotecan	Drugs which generally cause minimal nausea: • Alimta (pemetrexed) • Avastin (Bevacizumab) • Tarceva (erlotinib) • Erbitux (cetuximab) • Xalkori (crizotinib)

Drugs which can cause allergic reactions:
• Taxol (paclitaxel)
• Taxotere (docetaxel)
• Cytoxan (cyclophosphamide)
• Erbitux (cetuximab)

(continues)

Table 3 (continued)

Drugs which can cause numbness and tingling in the hands and feet (peripheral neuropathy):
- Taxol (paclitaxel)
- Taxotere (docetaxel)
- Cisplatin

Drugs which can cause hypertension:
- Avastin (bevacizumab)

Drugs which can cause visual changes:
- Xalkori (crizotinib)

* Please note that this is not a comprehensive list. Also, it does not include drugs which are used for the treatment of other types of cancer. Talk to your doctor about which drugs are best for you.

that this one mutation can drive a normal cell to become cancerous. Some mutations are targetable, meaning that their abnormal function can be inhibited by a drug scientists can design (**targetable mutation**). EGFR is a targetable mutation; scientists have designed drugs such as Tarceva to block the abnormal proteins made by a mutated EGFR. Thus, EGFR is both a driver mutation and a targetable one, which is why patients with an EGFR mutation often respond dramatically to Tarceva.

Most cancers are not caused by one specific driver mutation. They are caused by an accumulation of many mutations over time. The study of all the mutated genes in a tumor is called genomics. Since there are many, many genes that can become mutated, and these might or might not differ across tumors, analyzing all this data requires complicated computer programs designed by **biostatisticians** (statisticians who specialize in the study of the natural variations found in biology and the natural world). These programs often identify patterns (called **signatures**) in the mutations across tumors that can help

Targetable mutation

A mutation against which a drug can be made.

Biostatistician

A statistician who specializes in the study of the natural variations found in biology and the natural world.

Signatures

Patterns of expression of many genes or proteins, which is unique to that type of cancer.

identify which tumors are likely to be more aggressive than others and which are more likely to respond to which types of chemotherapy. A number of these genetic signatures have been identified; they are currently undergoing additional testing to determine which are likely to be the most accurate in predicting how a person might respond to any particular chemotherapy regimen.

56. What is personalized medicine?

Personalized medicine

Treatment of a patient not based upon where it arose, but upon the molecular characterization of the tumor, so that each patient will get a treatment designed specifically for them based upon the molecular characteristics of the tumor.

Another very active area of research for treatment of cancer is **personalized medicine**. Personalized medicine has been called, "The right drug for the right patient at the right time," and involves studying each patient's tumor and then designing the right treatment for that patient based upon the unique characteristics of that patient's tumor. For example, Tarceva and Xalkori work best in patients whose tumors have an EGFR mutation or an ALK fusion protein, respectively (see Question 45). Eventually, though, we would like to identify drugs that are targeted against many mutations, not just the EGFR mutation and EML-4/ALK fusion protein. By using techniques such as genomics (see Question 55), scientists hope to predict which chemotherapy the patient is more likely to be sensitive to or resistant to so that their physician can pick the right chemotherapy. Although we are not there yet, personalized medicine is the goal we are all striving for. By the time you read this, there will almost certainly be more drugs approved.

TREATMENT OF SCLC

57. What are the standard treatment options for my stage of SCLC?

Limited Stage

Limited Stage SCLC is potentially a curable disease. The optimal treatment consists of chemotherapy (usually four cycles) plus concurrent radiation therapy to the chest. However, as discussed in Question 54, this combination has significant side effects and probably should not be given to patients who are frail or who have bad lungs. Some physicians try to minimize the toxicity by giving the chemotherapy and radiation therapy sequentially instead of concurrently. In limited-stage SCLC, this is probably not as helpful as giving them at the same time. At least one study showed that if the radiation therapy is given twice per day for 12–15 days, instead of once per day for 20–25 fractions, patients are more likely to be cured.

Areas of Research and Clinical Trials (see also Questions 59 and 60)

Active areas of investigation include:

- What is the best dose of radiation therapy, and how frequently should it be delivered?
- What is the best chemotherapy?
- Are there any other treatments that can be administered after the chemotherapy is done to prevent the cancer from coming back?

Extensive-Stage SCLC

The principles behind chemotherapy for SCLC are the same as for NSCLC. Although patients with advanced, metastatic SCLC are rarely cured, they very often respond to chemotherapy, at least for a while. The typical chemotherapy regimens in the past have been a platin (carboplatin or cisplatin) plus etoposide (VP-16).

Areas of Research and Clinical Trials
(see also Questions 59 and 60)

An active area of clinical investigation is trying to identify types of chemotherapy regimens.

58. I have SCLC and my doctor has recommended prophylactic cranial irradiation (PCI). What is PCI, and how do I decide whether it is right for me?

Prophylactic cranial irradiation (**PCI**) is radiation to the brain with the intention of preventing the development of brain metastases. It is based on the premise that chemotherapy does not penetrate well into the brain so there could be micrometastases in the brain that have not been exposed to chemotherapy. PCI is recommended for SCLC patients who achieve complete **remission** following initial treatment because the brain is a common site of recurrence for SCLC. PCI reduces the incidence of brain metastases and improves both disease-free and overall survival for SCLC patients in complete remission.

The potential for mental impairment remains a primary concern for patients considering PCI. For most patients, this concern is unfounded. Although further research is

Prophylactic cranial irradiation (PCI)

Radiation to the brain with the intention of preventing the development of brain metastases.

Remission

Shrinkage of tumor in response to treatment. May be either complete (total disappearance of tumor) or partial (the tumor has shrunk, but has not gone away entirely).

needed, two large studies have shown that the long-term consequences of PCI on mental functioning are slight. The primary side effect of PCI is reversible hair loss.

If you are a candidate for PCI, you should discuss its pros and cons with both your oncologist and your radiation oncologist. An important question to ask is whether there is anything about you as an individual that puts you at risk for side effects. Although the risks from PCI are limited, certain patients can be more susceptible to side effects. Because SCLC patients face a high prospect of brain metastases—which are associated with disabling symptoms and early death—the decision to undergo PCI makes sense in most cases when considering both quality of life and survival.

INVESTIGATIVE/EXPERIMENTAL THERAPIES

59. What are clinical trials?

Clinical trials are research studies involving people (as opposed to preclinical studies which could involve animals). Through clinical trials, scientists learn how to fight cancer. There are many types of clinical trials (prevention, screening, treatment, quality of life) and questions that scientists can address by means of a clinical trial. The clinical trials process is designed to encourage the development of new drugs for cancer while protecting the volunteers who participate in the trials.

Participating in a clinical trial can sound scary. However, this is the only way any progress is made in the treatment of cancer. All drugs that we now have to

The clinical trials process is designed to encourage the development of new drugs for cancer while protecting the volunteers who participate in the trials.

treat cancer were developed through clinical trials, in which patients such as you participated. There are many reasons for participating in a clinical trial, but even if you do not benefit directly, the knowledge gained from your participation will help future lung cancer patients. The clinical trials process for a new cancer drug begins with an application by the study sponsor to the Food and Drug Administration (FDA) to conduct a clinical trial. The FDA is the U.S. government agency that approves new treatments for marketing and sale to the public. It provides oversight and approval for new drugs, new devices, new types of treatments, and new uses for established drugs, devices, and treatments. For most cancer trials, the study sponsor is either a pharmaceutical company, the National Cancer Institute, or one of its associated trial groups, such as the Eastern Cooperative Oncology Group [ECOG], the Southwestern Cooperative Oncology Group [SWOG], and ALLIANCE.

The study sponsor must demonstrate that testing of the drug in laboratory studies (in vitro studies, meaning in a Petrie dish or flask) and in animal studies (in vivo studies) showed promise with a reasonable expectation of safety in humans. After the investigational new drug (IND) application is approved, an investigational drug will usually undergo three phases of testing before it is eligible for final FDA approval:

- Phase I trials are designed to test the *safety* of the new drug. They usually involve a small number of patients (usually fewer than 50) who are given the drug in gradually increasing amounts to assess side effects and establish the most appropriate dose and schedule.
- Phase II trials determine how *effective* the drug is for treating a specific cancer. Phase II trials are usually

conducted in larger groups of people (anywhere from 25 to 200). If the drug looks like it might have activity in a certain tumor type, then a Phase III trial is conducted.

- Phase III trials are designed to test whether a new drug is better than the standard treatment for a specific cancer. Both the effectiveness of the drug and the amount and extent of side effects are compared. The number of people participating in Phase III trials can range from hundreds to thousands and typically involve dozens of hospitals in the United States and sometimes worldwide.

Phase III trials frequently employ a trial design called a **randomized controlled trial (RCT)**. In an RCT, the trial participants are randomly assigned (by chance, like the flip of a coin, although the randomization process is usually performed by a computer) to the treatment (experimental) group or the control (standard of care) group. You might hear these groups referred to as **arms**. The experimental arm receives the new treatment alone or the new treatment combined with standard treatment. The control arm receives the standard treatment. Assignment to one arm or another is not based on any medical information; it is random. Some trials are double-blinded, which means that neither the patients nor the doctors know who is in the experimental group and who is in the control group.

Randomization, control, and blinding are all scientific methods used to ensure that the trial results will not be biased in favor of one outcome or another. If clinical trials were not randomized, physicians might tend to refer all of one type of patient or another to a particular arm of the study. For example, if the medical

Randomized controlled trial (RCT)

A research study in which the participants are assigned by chance (using a computer) to separate groups that compare different treatments; a method used to prevent bias in research.

Arm of a clinical study

Treatment group to which a patient is assigned in a randomized clinical trial.

119

oncologist thinks a drug is particularly promising but is worried about side effects, given the option, he or she might decide to enter only the youngest patients into the investigational arm of the study and enter the older patients into the control arm, thereby possibly biasing the results.

One type of trial design that concerns many patients is a **placebo**-controlled trial. A placebo is a dummy or inactive substance (like a sugar pill) that is given to individuals in the control arm of certain trials. Some cancer patients avoid clinical trials for fear of getting a placebo. This fear is unfounded. *It is extremely rare that a placebo-only arm is used in a cancer treatment trial.* It is unethical to treat patients with a placebo when effective care is available, even if it is in the context of testing a promising new drug. The only circumstances in which a placebo-only arm is used in a treatment trial is if the standard of care for that type and stage of cancer is no treatment at all or in an RCT in which the two arms are standard chemo plus study drug or standard chemo plus placebo. In either case, both arms get standard chemo. *Your doctor will tell you if a study involves a placebo*, but you should ask in any case.

Placebo

An inactive substance (e.g., sugar pill). Placebos alone are rarely used in cancer trials.

60. How do I learn about clinical trials? How do I evaluate whether a trial is the right one for me?

Your first step should be to ask your oncologist whether a clinical trial might be appropriate for you. He or she might recommend a specific trial or trials and can discuss the pros and cons of your participation. You might also want to research clinical trials yourself to increase the chances that you have covered all of your options.

(This task can be delegated to a family member or friend if you are not up to the effort.) Your oncologist will be able to help you evaluate what you find. (For information on how to locate clinical trials, see the clinical trials locators listed in the Appendix.)

Before a study can begin, it must be reviewed by the Institutional Review Board (IRB) to make sure that the study is ethical (e.g., patients are not being denied an effective treatment) and as safe as possible. The IRB is an independent committee of the hospital that makes sure clinical studies meet ethical guidelines and that prospective participants are given all the information they need in order to make an **informed consent**.

If your doctor does not have access to clinical trials, the next step is to contact the principal investigator, or study coordinator, of the trial itself. He or she will evaluate your eligibility for the trial by reviewing the inclusion criteria (for example, type and stage of lung cancer) and exclusion criteria (for example, some studies might exclude patients with kidney disease for safety reasons or require potential participants to have had no prior chemotherapy). Eligibility criteria are used to protect participants and also to ensure that the study participants are alike in certain ways so that trial results will be more reliable.

After it has been determined that you are a potential candidate for the trial, the informed consent process begins. The process of informed consent is designed to protect your interests and safety as a trial participant in a scientific experiment by giving you the information you need to make an informed decision about whether to participate. The process begins when the investigator or study coordinator explains the trial to you. He or she

Informed consent

A process that provides potential participants in a clinical trial the information they need to make an informed decision about whether or not to participate.

will describe the purpose of the study, why you are eligible, how many people are participating, the procedures and design of the trial, the anticipated risks (which could include physical, financial, psychological, and legal risks in addition to any potential risks to your privacy/confidentiality), the costs of the trial, if any, as well as alternatives that might be open to you other than the trial. Your rights as a trial participant should be made clear: Your participation in a clinical trial is voluntary; you are free to stop the study at any time; and there will be no penalty if you decide to stop (e.g., your doctor will not be angry at you). Before you sign the informed consent document, ask your doctor who will cover the costs of the trial, including the costs of treating any unexpected side effects. Be sure you understand everything and that you discuss it with whomever you trust to help you with your medical decisions.

Before you sign the informed consent document, ask your doctor who will cover the costs of the trial, including the costs of treating any unexpected side effects. Be sure you understand everything and that you discuss it with whomever you trust to help you with your medical decisions.

There are many good reasons why you might consider participating in a clinical trial: you could have run out of the standard treatments available to treat your lung cancer; you might feel that standard therapies don't have much to offer you and that a potential new drug holds more promise; you might feel that you will get better care in a clinical trial; or you might want to help patients who come after you. Whatever your motive(s), you should be sure you understand the differences (in terms of risks, benefits, and practical considerations, such as time and cost) between a clinical trial and your other options. Only then can you make a truly informed decision.

ALTERNATIVE THERAPIES

61. What is alternative medicine?

Alternative medicine generally refers to therapies developed outside of mainstream medicine and used in place of standard, clinically proven therapies. Some of these therapies are touted as cures for cancer, with little or no scientific information to support them. It is often impossible to establish the reliability of individual testimonials, locate scientific research on alternative therapies, or verify the credentials of an alternative medicine practitioner. Unproved alternative therapies are often promoted and sold by the same person, a charlatan who attempts to take advantage of vulnerable cancer patients. Insurance does not cover these types of alternative treatments. The cost of alternative medicine can be significant in terms of dollars, and in wasted time and energy. Most importantly, they can be dangerous to your health.

On the other hand, alternative medicine can also describe traditional medical systems, such as Traditional Chinese Medicine (TCM) or Ayurveda (from India). Although these systems have been in use for centuries, they have not been studied with the same scientific rigor as Western medicine. Because of this lack of data, many in the Western medical community view these alternative systems with skepticism and resistance.

When alternative methods are used in addition to conventional therapy, it is often referred to as complementary medicine. Although complementary medicine can include approaches such as herbal therapies, the term often refers to methods such as acupuncture and mind/body techniques (guided imagery, meditation) that are aimed at improving side effects and symptoms rather than curing disease. Complementary methods can range from nutritional supplements and herbal therapies, to hypnotism and biofeedback, to art therapy and spiritual practices.

Complementary and alternative medicine (CAM)

Therapies developed outside of mainstream medicine and used in place of standard, clinically proven therapies.

There has long been a disconnect between patients and doctors with regard to the use of **complementary and alternative medicine** (**CAM**). A significant percentage of patients use some type of complementary therapy but do not share this information with their doctors. Some patients feel that their doctors would not be receptive; others see no reason to tell their doctors. Doctors often fail to ask patients about their use of complementary medicine. For some doctors this could reflect a bias against alternative methods or a lack of expertise; for others, it might reflect an ignorance or lack of concern about the prevalence of CAM use among patients. Poor communication on CAM issues can compromise patient care. The good news is that there is more ongoing scientific research into CAM therapies, thereby encouraging awareness and dialogue on CAM issues. The National Institutes of Health has established the National Center for Complementary and Alternative Medicine (NCCAM), dedicated to encouraging research and distributing accurate information on CAM therapies. The National Cancer Institute's Office of Cancer Complementary and Alternative Medicine (OCCAM) supports the NCCAM mandate, focusing specifically on CAM for cancer.

- If you are interested in pursuing alternative therapies, first check the NCCAM (*www.nccam.nih.gov*) and OCCAM (*www.cancer.gov/cam/*) websites to see if there is evidence of safety and effectiveness. This should be done for both alternative and complementary treatments. You will find comprehensive fact sheets and summaries on individual therapies (e.g., antineoplastons, acupuncture, coenzyme Q10, dietary supplements) with links to both CAM clinical trials and CAM scientific literature. Another valuable resource for checking the reliability of alternative therapies marketed to cancer patients is Quackwatch (*www.quackwatch.com*). Quackwatch reviews the evidence and provides critiques of these therapies and should be consulted prior to undergoing any alternative treatment. Your doctor can help you to evaluate what you find in your research and advise you on whether a therapy or method might make sense for you.

- It is crucial to understand that herbal treatments and dietary supplements (vitamins) are not regulated by the Food and Drug Administration (FDA), and therefore, any claims about anti-tumor efficacy have not been proven or reproduced by independent investigators. There are also reasons to be concerned about quality control, as well as issues of safety and effectiveness in these substances that you might consider safe. The best policy is to discuss the possible consequences of taking these substances with your doctor before you take them.

- Check the credentials of your CAM practitioner carefully. Ask for information on education, training, and membership in professional organizations. Complementary therapies abound. Some patients find that activities such as meditation, guided imagery, yoga, and tai chi help them to relieve pain, stress, anxiety, and increase their quality of life. There is little scientific data, however, that they are helpful in controlling cancer. For further information on the complementary therapies available to you, check with your hospital's patient center or contact a cancer support organization such as CancerCare or the Wellness Community.

TREATMENT OF SPECIAL POPULATIONS AND CONDITIONS

62. I am 78 years old. Am I too old for chemo? Will it be too tough on me? Are there particular considerations for treatment of elderly lung cancer patients?

Age alone should not prevent you from receiving treatment for lung cancer.

Age alone should not prevent you from receiving treatment for lung cancer. Elderly patients can undergo chemotherapy, radiation, and/or surgery if their overall health allows them to withstand the stress of treatment. Generally speaking, older patients tolerate treatment as well as their younger counterparts, providing they are healthy. Your doctor will determine your ability to undergo treatment by assessing your level of function (called performance status—see Question 34) and any coexisting medical problems that could complicate some treatments. These circumstances are often a primary consideration when determining treatment options. However, it is important to recognize that your overall condition is a better predictor of your ability to tolerate treatment than is your chronological age.

When a chemotherapy drug is given alone as treatment, it is called monotherapy. Several chemotherapy drugs have been studied for use as monotherapies in elderly lung cancer patients with encouraging outcomes and fewer side effects than the standard multi-drug regimens. These chemotherapies include vinorelbine, docetaxel, Alimta, gemcitabine, and paclitaxel. Although elderly patients with good performance status can undergo standard chemotherapy regimens involving multiple drugs, patients with less-than-optimal performance status are frequently ineligible for regimens involving multiple adverse effects. Single-drug regimens can be a good choice for these patients, offering less toxicity without sacrificing effectiveness. Some of the newer, experimental treatment agents might also be appropriate for patients with poor performance status because many of these agents target tumor cells and leave normal cells unaffected, resulting in fewer and less toxic side effects.

For lobectomy or wedge resections, age alone is not a risk factor, and elderly patients who are otherwise healthy should not be denied these surgical options based on chronological age. When surgery involves removal of the entire lung (pneumonectomy), however, there is a considerable risk of post-op complications and death over the age of 70. Pneumonectomy in the elderly should be undertaken with great caution and consideration. When feasible, video-assisted thoracoscopic surgery (VATS) or robotic surgery offers a safer, less invasive alternative to traditional open procedures for all lung cancer patients. Alternative treatment options are available for patients who are judged to be medically inoperable (due to poor performance status or coexisting illnesses). For example, radiotherapy (with curative intent) has been used in elderly patients who are not surgical candidates, but who have potentially curable early stage NSCLC.

If you are elderly with lung cancer, you should be alert to any age bias on the part of your doctor—it is both inappropriate and substandard care to receive less aggressive treatment solely because of your age. Elderly patients who are in good health and have a good performance status face no greater risks from standard treatments based on their age alone. For those elderly patients with compromised performance status and/or limiting illness, there could be alternative treatment options available.

Communication with your doctor is essential to learning all of your treatment options. Only then can you make an informed decision based on what is right for you—whatever your age.

63. My doctor told me that I have developed brain metastases. What are my treatment options?

There are several ways to treat brain metastases, and your doctor will advise you about which treatments might be appropriate in your individual case.

There are several ways to treat brain metastases, and your doctor will advise you about which treatments might be appropriate in your individual case. Traditional surgery could occasionally be used to remove a brain metastasis, particularly if there is only one metastasis and the tumor elsewhere in your body is under relatively good control. More likely, you will be treated with radiation. Whole brain radiation might be used to shrink or eradicate the tumors if you have numerous small metastases. Stereotactic radiosurgery (pinpoint radiation; also known as Gamma Knife or Cyber Knife, depending upon the machine being used) could be used alone or in conjunction with whole brain radiation when there are only a few small metastases. In some cases, chemotherapy used to treat primary brain tumors has been used in patients with brain metastases, but there is no evidence that these treatments are effective in prolonging survival for lung cancer patients.

64. How are bone metastases treated?

If your lung cancer has metastasized to your bones, treatment will be aimed at reducing pain and strengthening the bone to reduce the risk of fractures. Common sites of bone metastasis are the vertebrae, ribs, hips, leg, and arm bones. Traditional radiation therapy to the involved area is effective for reducing pain. Occasionally, if the tumor has weakened the bone to the verge of breaking, surgery could be recommended to remove the bone tumor and stabilize the bone to prevent future breakage. Another method for treating bone metastases is drug therapy using a class of drugs called bisphosphonates, such as Zometa (zoledronic acid) or XGEVA (denosumab). These drugs are not chemotherapy. That is, they do not kill cancer cells directly. Instead, these drugs strengthen bone, thus reducing the chance of developing bone metastasis.

EVALUATING TREATMENT OPTIONS AND OUTCOMES

65. How do I decide on a treatment plan when I am faced with multiple options?

This is a difficult question. Talk with your doctor, and make sure you know all of your treatment options and that you understand the differences among them. Carefully weigh the pros and cons of each treatment, and evaluate your priorities. Many factors can influence your decision. These could include treatment survival rates, side effects and quality-of-life concerns, cost, time commitment, travel, and so on. If, for example, being home as much as possible is one of your top priorities, you would be less likely to choose a daily intravenous treatment than one that requires coming to the hospital only once every 3 weeks.

Your doctor will advise you on your options and make treatment recommendations based upon his or her medical experience and training and on what he or she knows about you, your tumor, and your priorities. Many patients feel pressured and/or overwhelmed with having to make the decision and prefer to follow their doctor's recommendation. Other people like to be more actively involved in the decision-making process. Whatever your preference, the doctor-patient relationship is a critical component of the process. If you communicate effectively with your doctor regarding what you want from your treatment, it will allow him or her to provide you with optimal treatment advice.

66. How do I know if my treatment is working? What is the difference between partial response and complete response? What is a remission?

Partial response

A decrease in the size of a tumor, or in the extent of cancer in the body, in response to treatment. Also called partial remission.

Complete response

The disappearance of all signs of cancer in response to treatment. This does not always mean the cancer has been cured. Also called complete remission.

A remission is another word for response. For some reason hematologists tend to use the word remission for leukemia and lymphoma, while oncologists (solid tumor doctors) tend to use the word response when talking about cancers such as lung cancer. A **partial response** (or **partial remission**) is defined as an approximate 30% shrinkage of the tumor as determined by X-ray, CT scan, or physical exam. A **complete response** (or **complete remission**) is total disappearance of the tumor. Note, however, that neither a partial nor a complete response necessarily translates into cure. It is not uncommon for a patient to have a temporary response, meaning that the tumor initially shrinks with chemotherapy but then starts to grow at some point. Probably, the chemotherapy killed off the sensitive cancer cells, leaving behind a population of cancer cells that were more resistant to chemotherapy and which eventually started to grow.

In the past, the official way to tell whether the treatment is working is to get another scan and see whether the tumor is shrinking. Many patients can tell even before the scan is taken because their symptoms from the cancer improve as the tumor shrinks. However, many chemotherapy regimens don't actually shrink the tumor—they stop it from growing (stable disease).

67. What if my disease has remained stable during treatment?

If your disease is stable, that's good! It means you and your doctor are achieving your goal—stopping the cancer from growing. There are many cases in which a patient's tumor never shrank according to a CT scan but never grew either. Presumably, in these situations the cancer cells must have been killed by the treatment but never disintegrated enough to make it look like the tumor was shrinking. Another possibility is that the tumor on the scan could now contain a lot of scar tissue that formed from the treatment.

68. What happens if my disease recurs? How is recurrence treated? Is it possible to survive a recurrence of lung cancer?

Recurrence is something that every lung cancer patient fears. If you have experienced a recurrence, do not despair. Although cure following a recurrence is rare, long-term survival is not impossible. Try not to let yourself become overwhelmed or paralyzed by this news—it is almost always the case that you will have treatment options that can increase your survival. Discuss these options with your doctor, including clinical trials, of which there are many (see Questions 59 and 60). Follow the same decision-making process as you did when you were initially diagnosed. Weigh the pros and cons of each option. Make informed decisions. When dealing with recurrent lung cancer or lung cancer that does not respond to treatment, it is especially important that you communicate with your doctor regarding your changing needs and priorities.

Ask yourself how aggressive you want to be. Each time the tumor grows after treatment, it tends to become slightly more resistant to chemotherapy. You might find that quality of life becomes a greater concern if your disease continues to progress despite treatment. However, if aggressively attacking the tumor as much as possible is something you want to do, advocate for yourself. Ask your physician very specifically what the alternative treatments are. If he or she cannot provide any, seek a second opinion at an academic cancer center (see Questions 21 and 22).

Chemotherapy Drugs for Lung Cancer

Chemotherapy recommendations vary depending on whether you have NSCLC or SCLC. New types of chemotherapy are under development all the time; this book is not meant to discuss them in detail. (See Part 7 for Side Effects.)

NSCLC

First-line therapy
Initial treatment.

For NSCLC, **first-line therapy** (e.g., initial treatment) will often consist of two drugs, one of which is usually a platinum (cisplatin or carboplatin). Available non-platinum drugs include docetaxel (Taxotere), gemcitabine (Gemzar), paclitaxel (Taxol), pemetrexed (Alimta), and vinorelbine (Navelbine). In general, the two-drug regimens used for NSCLC have roughly the same success rate in shrinking the tumor and prolonging life. However, they do have different side effects, schedules of administration, and cost so many oncologists will base their decision on which one to recommend based on these factors. Bevacizumab (Avastin) is often added for those patients who do not have squamous cell carcinoma and who have not coughed up any blood (**hemoptysis**).

Should lung cancer progress during or following initial chemotherapy, oncologists will often recommend additional therapy. Docetaxel (Taxotere) and pemetrexed (Alimta) are two chemotherapy drugs that have been approved in the United States for **second-line treatment** of NSCLC. Oncologists sometimes use gemcitabine (Gemzar) if the patient did not receive it previously. Erlotinib (Tarceva), a targeted therapy, has been approved for both second and third-line treatment. Your oncologist can tell you which option makes sense for your situation.

SCLC
For SCLC, first-line therapy is often etoposide (VP-16) and either cisplatin or carboplatin. Second-line therapy for SCLC could include the following additional regimens and drugs: cyclophosphamide, doxorubicin, vincristine, carboplatin, etoposide (VP-16), ifosfamide, and topotecan.

How to Learn More About Chemotherapy Drugs
It is best to discuss your chemotherapy alternatives with your oncologist because new chemotherapy drugs and regimens are constantly under development. Your oncologist will be able to advise you on the likely side

Hemoptysis
Coughing up blood.

Second-line treatment
Treatment method(s) used following an initial treatment that either does not stop cancer progression or stops it only temporarily.

effects. If you are interested in further information about chemotherapy drugs, you can consult the following resources.

Clinical Research

To learn more about the effectiveness of lung cancer chemotherapies, you can search the medical literature via PubMed at: *www.pubmed.org*. Enter the term "lung cancer" (use quotes) and the drug name in the search box separated by the word "AND" in all capital letters. For example: "lung cancer" AND carboplatin.

You can further refine your search by clicking on Chose Additional Features, which allows you to limit your search in various ways, such as by date, language, and type of publication.

Side Effects

Ask your oncologist about the potential side effects of your chemotherapy regimen. He or she will be able to tell you what to expect and what to do if you experience side effects. MEDLINEplus, the National Library of Medicine's consumer health website, is also an excellent source of detailed information on chemotherapies and other drugs. For each drug, MEDLINEplus lists the brand name(s); a description; things to know before using the drug, such as allergy or pregnancy considerations; and a list of common, less common, and rare side effects. To access the MEDLINEplus drug database, go to *www.medlineplus.gov* and click on Drugs & Supplements. *Gail Wilkes's The Consumers Guide to Cancer Drugs* (Jones and Bartlett Learning, 2003) provides similar information on chemotherapy drug side effects.

To learn more about the effectiveness of lung cancer chemotherapies, you can search the medical literature via PubMed at www.pubmed.org.

Side Effects of Chemotherapy

What are the common side effects of chemotherapy?

What are blood counts, and what should I know about them?

Why am I always exhausted? What can I do for fatigue? Will the fatigue go away after my treatment is over?

More . . .

69. *What are the common side effects of chemotherapy?*

The particular side effects you experience will depend on which chemotherapy drugs you receive and your individual response. You should ask your oncologist or oncology nurse for information on the common side effects associated with your chemotherapy regimen. You need to be aware of how to manage the common effects and under what circumstances you should call your oncologist. Some patients find it helpful to keep a journal during chemotherapy treatment to record the dates, times, and duration of symptoms, along with descriptive information. The more accurate you can be in reporting your symptoms to your oncologist, the better care you will receive.

The more accurate you can be in reporting your symptoms to your oncologist, the better care you will receive.

Although there are numerous side effects associated with chemotherapy, it is important to remember that no one gets all of them. In fact, most patients experience relatively few side effects. Common chemotherapy side effects include:

- Fatigue. Fatigue is one of the most commons side effects of chemotherapy, although for most patients, it is relatively mild. It tends to be at its worst for about 1 week following chemotherapy. Many lung cancer patients are able to continue working, although many cut back to part time. If your fatigue is overwhelming, tell your doctor because there could be something else going on.
- Hair loss (alopecia). Please note that not all lung cancer chemotherapy drugs cause hair loss. Ask your doctor (see Table 3).
- Mild nausea and, rarely, vomiting

- Drop in blood counts (white blood cells, red blood cells, or platelets). This is called myelosuppression and is a potentially serious side effect of chemotherapy (see Question 70).

Less common effects:

- Infection
- Skin and nail problems
- Loss of appetite
- Peripheral neuropathy
- Allergic reactions
- Sexual effects: desire, fertility, hormonal balance
- Oral effects: sore mouth and gums, changes in taste
- Gastrointestinal effects: diarrhea and constipation

70. What are blood counts, and what should I know about them?

To monitor the effects of chemotherapy on your blood count (hematologic effects), your oncologist will order a test called a complete blood count (CBC). A CBC counts each type of blood cell. Blood tests are usually performed prior to chemo and can be performed when counts are predicted to be low. Low blood counts could cause your chemotherapy treatments to be postponed or modified until the passage of time brings them back to safe levels. There are also medications your doctor can prescribe.

You should be aware of the following conditions caused by the effect of chemotherapy on blood counts.

Neutropenia

Low white blood cell count.

Neutrophil

A type of white blood cell that attacks bacteria.

Nadir

Lowest measured value; period of low blood counts.

Colony-stimulating factors

Substances that stimulate bone marrow to increase production of blood cells; also referred to as growth factors.

Neutropenia: a low white blood cell (WBC) count. White blood cells fight infection in your body. **Neutrophils** are one type of white blood cell that attacks bacteria. If your neutrophil count (called absolute neutrophil count, or ANC) drops to low levels, you are at higher risk of infection, including serious, potentially life-threatening side effects such as pneumonia. Neutropenia can be a dangerous condition for a cancer patient because infections in neutrapenic patients tend to be more severe than in other individuals and might require hospitalization for IV antibiotics. If your counts indicate that your neutrophils are significantly below normal (a period called the **nadir** that usually occurs 10–14 days following treatment), you should avoid situations that might increase your risk of infection. For example, you can wash your hands frequently, avoid crowds (shopping malls, movie theaters, classrooms) or exposure to individuals with illness, and avoid eating uncooked and undercooked foods. Neutropenia can be treated with drugs called **colony-stimulating factors** (such as Neupogen, Neulasta, and Leukine) that cause your bone marrow to increase the number of white blood cells. If you experience fever, chills, sweats, or other symptoms of infection while getting chemo, you should contact your oncologist's office promptly.

Although neutropenia can occur with almost all types of chemotherapy, the chemotherapy commonly used in lung cancer does not usually result in neutropenia that is so severe, or of such a long duration, that patients come down with an infection. Fortunately, the chances of coming down with an infection are relatively low for lung cancer patients compared to other cancer patients who get different types of chemotherapy.

Anemia: a low **red blood cell** (**RBC**) count. Your red blood cells carry oxygen to your body. A low RBC count means that there is not enough oxygen in your blood—you are anemic. Your oncologist might refer to a low **hematocrit** (a measure of the number of RBCs in your blood) or a low **hemoglobin** (a protein in RBCs), which are two specific measures for anemia. If you become anemic, you could experience fatigue, weakness, and dizziness; headache and shortness of breath can also be symptoms of anemia. In some cases, a blood transfusion might be necessary to restore your RBC count to safe levels. In the past, physicians often gave a medication called erythropoietin (Epo; ProCrit; Aranesp) to increase the number of RBCs. However, these medications have become very controversial, since they have recently been found to cause blood clots, and, in some cancers, increase the risk of death. Because of this the FDA has significantly restricted the use of these medications in cancer patients.

Thrombocytopenia: low platelet levels. Platelets are a type of blood cell that helps stop bleeding. Patients with low levels of platelets might experience bruising or bleeding (e.g., nosebleeds, bleeding gums, intestinal bleeding). If necessary, patients can also undergo a platelet transfusion to increase the platelet count. Although there is a drug called thrombopoietin that can help prevent thrombocytopenia, it has so many side effects that it is rarely used for lung cancer patients. Fortunately, the chemotherapy commonly given for lung cancer rarely causes significant thrombocytopenia.

The effect of chemotherapy on blood counts varies widely among patients depending on the chemotherapy

---

SIDE EFFECTS OF CHEMOTHERAPY

Anemia

Low red blood cell count; may cause tiredness, weakness, and shortness of breath.

Red blood cell (RBC)

The most common type of blood cell and the body's principal means of delivering oxygen to the body tissues via the blood.

Hematocrit

The proportion of the blood that consists of red blood cells.

Hemoglobin

The oxygen-carrying protein in the red blood cells.

Thrombocytopenia

Low counts of platelets that could result in bruising and/or bleeding.

regimen and on the patient's individual response. For example, cisplatin and premetrexed (Alimta) rarely cause any significant drop in the counts, while gemcitabine and carboplatin cause thrombocytopenia. Taxol, Taxotere, and Navelbine cause neutropenia. The targeted agents, such as Avastin, Tarceva, Xalkori, and Erbitux are targeted at pathways found only in cancer so they rarely cause significant myelosuppression. Some patients experience only mild drops in blood counts and have few related symptoms. If you are aware of the possible effects (and associated symptoms) of chemotherapy on your blood, you will be able to identify potential problems, alert your doctor in a timely manner, and receive more effective treatment.

71. Why am I always exhausted? What can I do for fatigue? Will the fatigue go away after my treatment is over?

There are a number of possible reasons for fatigue, particularly while on chemotherapy. One that was popularized due to many commercials and magazine ads is fatigue due to anemia from the chemotherapy. A blood test ordered by your doctor should indicate if your red blood cell (RBC) count is low enough to be the cause of your fatigue. If you are anemic, your doctor might order a blood transfusion or a medication called erythropoietin (Procrit, Epo, Aranesp). However, these medications have become much more regulated recently due to their tendency to cause blood clots. In some types of cancer, there is also data to suggest that they could shorten a cancer patient's life. For these reasons, doctors are currently able to prescribe these medications only under strict conditions. However, he or she might order a blood transfusion instead.

Another possible reason for fatigue is depression. Depression can manifest in many ways, not just an overwhelming feeling of sadness. Patients can feel despair, discouragement, lack of interest in activities they once enjoyed, change in sleeping patterns or eating patterns, and fatigue. Although anyone with cancer might experience some of these feelings some of the time, a person is clinically depressed when the depression is of such a magnitude that he or she is not able to enjoy any activities that normally bring pleasure. If you feel this might be a possibility, talk with your doctor. (See Question 80 for additional discussion of depression.)

In many cases, however, it is not easy to identify and correct the cause of fatigue. Chemotherapy and radiation are tiring—be prepared for it. Manage it by getting the rest you need and by being proactive about reducing your activities. Consider cutting back at work to part time, if at all possible. Find out in advance what your company's policy is regarding medical leaves of absence. Pamper yourself—accept help from friends. Don't worry about a messy house. Explain to your family that your body is undergoing a change and that you will not be able to do as much for the next several months. If your family has a hard time accepting this, have them come to an appointment and discuss this with your doctor or social worker.

SIDE EFFECTS OF CHEMOTHERAPY

72. I have heard stories from patients who underwent chemotherapy years ago and had terrible nausea and vomiting. Will I have a similar experience?

Almost certainly you will not. The good news is that a new class of antiemetic drugs that is much more effective in preventing nausea and vomiting has been developed over the past decade. This class of antiemetics, called HT3 blockers, can be given orally or intravenously. These drugs have had a major impact on the ability of doctors to administer—and patients to tolerate—chemotherapy. A number of these are available (Kytril, Anzamet, and Emend, to name a few). Even the worst chemotherapy drugs these days often result in only some queasiness and loss of appetite for a day or 2. Vomiting is much less common than it has been in the past. The bad news is that these drugs can be very expensive, particularly if taken orally, because some insurance companies do not pay for oral medications. Most oncologists will give these medications intravenously with chemotherapy, making chemotherapy considerably more tolerable than it was in the past. However, everyone is different. If you are unusually sensitive to the nausea side effects of chemotherapy and have problems with repeated vomiting episodes, call your doctor or nurse. Do not wait for your next visit! It is important not to become dehydrated—this will only make you feel worse, which will result in less fluid intake, and start a downhill spiral. If you call while you are having the problem, your doctor or nurse will alter your medications and might even have you come to the office to receive fluids and antiemetics intravenously, which can help significantly.

Another drug very good at controlling nausea is the steroid dexamethasone or Decadron. Dexamethasone is much cheaper than the HT3 blockers and is often given in combination with them. Side effects include elevation of the blood glucose for several days so people with diabetes should take it with caution.

73. Will I lose my hair during chemotherapy or radiation? What can I do to make the experience more tolerable?

Hair loss, also known as alopecia, is one of the most common and dreaded of all cancer treatment side effects. Hair loss is difficult because it takes away your normal appearance and provides a constant reminder that you have cancer. You could feel that you are not yourself without your hair, and you might be uncomfortable or self-conscious around other people, even your family. It helps to remember that in the vast majority of cases, treatment-related hair loss is temporary, and there are things you can do to minimize the emotional and physical impact of losing your hair.

Some chemotherapy drugs are more likely to cause hair loss than others (see Table 3). Whether or not a drug causes hair loss is not an indication of how effective it is against killing cancer cells. Often, when faced with a new diagnosis of lung cancer, patients are so anxious to start treatment they forget to discuss some of the side effects with their doctor. If hair loss is important to you, tell your doctor! He or she can usually devise treatment plans less likely to cause hair loss without compromising how well the treatment works against the cancer.

Hair loss occurs because, in addition to cancer cells, both chemotherapy and radiation treatment adversely affect hair follicles and other fast-growing normal cells. With chemotherapy, your hair loss can range from a noticeable thinning, to patchy loss, to complete hair loss—or your hair might not be affected at all. The degree and nature of your hair loss will depend primarily on the type and amount of chemotherapy you are receiving. Your oncologist will be able to tell you what to expect, although to some extent the amount of hair loss varies from person to person. If you do lose your hair, it will begin to grow back about a month after your last treatment and take several more months to grow back fully. You shouldn't be surprised if the hair that grows back is a different texture or color than your normal hair. A change in texture is common, although over time your hair will most likely return to its original state. Extended chemotherapy treatments could also result in the loss of your body hair.

This phenomenon presents additional challenges—for example, your nose will run frequently and sweat will drip in your eyes. For some people, the loss of eyebrows and eyelashes is more disturbing than the loss of hair, which is more easily camouflaged.

Cranial irradiation

The exposure of the head to roentgen rays or other forms of radioactivity for therapeutic or preventive purposes.

With radiation, you will experience hair loss only in the area that is irradiated. Patients who receive **cranial irradiation** (radiation to the brain) almost always have total alopecia. Your hair will usually grow back, although it might be thinner than it was previously. Your hair loss could be permanent if you receive high doses of radiation.

There are several things you can do to make your experience with treatment-related hair loss more tolerable. The first thing is to prepare ahead of time. You might want to cut your hair to a short style to make the transition less traumatic. If your hair loss begins with a gradual thinning, you can reduce the rate of loss by avoiding the use of heat (curling irons, hair dryers, hot rollers) or chemicals (bleach, dyes, perms, harsh shampoos) and by using a soft brush. If your hair begins to fall out in clumps, you might find it easier and less upsetting to just shave your head at that point.

If you are planning on wearing a wig, try to get one before you start chemotherapy so you will have it when you need it. Your oncology nurse or social worker might be able to help you locate a wig shop that caters to the needs of cancer patients. Be sure to ask about the different types of wigs available and the advantages and disadvantages of each. It is possible to take your wig to your hairdresser and have it styled to look like your natural hair so that when you do make the transition, it will be less noticeable. Wigs vary greatly in cost depending on the quality of the wig you select, but your oncologist can give you a prescription for a hair prosthesis that will cover some or all of the expense if you have insurance coverage. A wig is considered a deductible medical expense. If you cannot afford a wig, the American Cancer Society, CancerCare, and other cancer organizations provide wigs free of charge to those in need.

There is a wealth of choices for head coverings, including hats, scarves, and turbans. The American Cancer Society's Tender Loving Care catalog (*www.tlccatalog.org* or (800) 850-9445) is a wonderful resource for these items and others designed specifically to hide hair loss. Keep in mind that there are no rules for what you should wear on your head, if anything, and you should do whatever is most comfortable for you.

Another excellent resource for learning to cope with hair loss is the Look Good...Feel Better program (*www.lookgoodfeelbetter.org*) that is sponsored by the American Cancer Society and certain other nonprofit organizations. The program offers workshops in skin care, makeup, hair and nail care, and the use of wigs and headwear. They provide many useful tips for coping with head and body hair loss and provide free samples to take home. If you are not comfortable attending the program yourself, a friend or relative can go for you, or you can ask to see the program video.

Understanding that your hair loss is temporary will help you to get through this tough time.

Understanding that your hair loss is temporary will help you to get through this tough time.

74. I have numbness and pain in my fingers and toes that my doctor calls peripheral neuropathy. Is there an effective treatment for this condition?

Peripheral neuropathy occurs when peripheral nerves (the nerves located outside of the brain and spinal chord) are damaged. This condition can be caused by your tumor, but, in most lung cancer patients, it is usually caused by certain chemotherapy drugs, such as paclitaxel (Taxol) or cisplatin. Symptoms of peripheral neuropathy could include feelings of pins and needles, numbness, and burning in the hands, feet, and legs. Motor problems, such as dropping things or problems walking, can also result from peripheral neuropathy. Sometimes a drug called Neurontin (gabapentin) can help, but this drug also has its side effects, such as fatigue. Some patients report that exercise helps with peripheral neuropathy and improves quality of life. In general, although the neuropathy rarely goes away completely, it can slowly improve with time. See the Appendix for resources to consult if you experience peripheral neuropathy.

75. What can I do about the rash I got with drugs like Tarceva or Erbitux?

Rash is one of the most common side effects for patients taking drugs like Tarceva or Erbitux (the drugs which inhibit the EGFR pathway; see Question 45) and can range from mild to severe. Typically, the rash, which often looks like acne, develops about 8 to 10 days after the start of treatment and affects areas above the waist. The rash is believed to be due to an inflammatory response as a result of EGFR inhibition in skin tissue and can be controlled with mild antibiotics. In most cases, the rash will improve with treatment. Tarceva rash is typically mild to moderate and can be managed by treating the rash and symptoms with a hydrocortisone cream or clindamycin gel. In some cases doxycycline or minocycline could also be prescribed.

Cases of severe rash can be unpleasant enough for some people to consider discontinuing treatment; however, recent data suggests that moderate to severe rash might be related to a better clinical outcome. You and your doctor should discuss the pros and cons and together determine when and if it becomes severe enough to reduce the dose or interrupt the treatment.

76. Will treatment for lung cancer make me infertile? Will it affect my sex life?

Chemotherapy can cause temporary or permanent infertility. If you think you might want to have children in the future, it is extremely important that you discuss this issue with your doctor prior to treatment. Factors that could affect fertility include the type of drug(s), the amount of drug you receive, the duration, and your individual response. Your doctor can advise you on your likelihood of infertility and on any steps that you might take to preserve your ability to have children—such as freezing your eggs or sperm for future use. Your doctor can also tell you whether you have any treatment alternatives that will not threaten your ability to have children. Radiation and surgery for lung cancer usually do not affect fertility, although to the extent that they reduce lung function, they could affect a woman's ability to carry a child. Some of the treatment agents currently in clinical trials for lung cancer do not affect fertility; however, the fertility effects of some experimental agents might be unknown. There could be nothing you can do to preserve your ability to have children in the face of lung cancer. If you share your concerns about this vital issue with your doctor, then he or she will be better able to advise you on your choices and help you to make these difficult decisions.

Your lung cancer impacts all aspects of your life, including your sexuality. A lung cancer diagnosis could affect how you feel about yourself sexually and how your partner feels about you. The pain, fatigue, shortness of breath, and other effects of cancer and its treatment affect you physically and emotionally and most likely will have a negative impact on your sex life. Communication is your best ally for combating this undesirable side effect. Communicate with your partner to let him or her know how you are feeling and how your disease and its treatment are affecting you sexually. Ask questions of your partner to be sure that he or she is expressing his or her feelings about changes that might be occurring as a result of your cancer. Discuss what you can do to accommodate these changes, such as making mental adjustments or devising alternatives to compensate for physical limitations. Talk to your doctor to learn whether there are things you can do to improve the symptoms that are interfering with your usual sex life. If your sexual relationship with your partner becomes a source of stress or concern, do not hesitate to discuss this with your doctor. Emotions and fear about cancer can cause you or your partner to make wrong assumptions or act in ways that result in hurt feelings. They can contribute to poor communication or worsen problems that existed prior to your lung cancer diagnosis. If you and your partner are having difficulties dealing with how your cancer is affecting your sex life, do not hesitate to seek professional counseling.

77. What can I do if I have lost my appetite?

Loss of appetite is a problem for many cancer patients and often a major source of concern for family members. Some things to consider include:

- Eat small meals more frequently (rather than three meals per day).
- Although it is always best to eat a well-balanced meal, for cancer patients who are struggling with loss of appetite, consuming calories is probably more important. Concentrate on eating high-calorie and

high-protein foods. A variety of nutritional supplements are available; many patients feel that they taste better cold and can mix them with ice cream or pudding.

- Talk to a nutritionist.
- There is a medication called Megace (megestrol) that can help stimulate the appetite. Ask your doctor about it.

78. Are there long-term, permanent side effects from treatment?

Your cancer treatments cause side effects. Many of these effects are temporary and disappear shortly after your treatment ends. Others might persist for years before resolving, and some might never go away completely. There are also late effects associated with treatment—effects that can appear up to years following cessation of treatment. It helps to be aware of these long-term and late effects so that you can incorporate this information into your treatment decisions. It is also important that you bring up these issues with your doctor so that, if at all possible, steps can be taken to eliminate or improve these treatment-related problems. As cancer patients are surviving longer, more is becoming known about these long-term health issues. This increased awareness helps patients to recognize these effects and to seek treatment and/or proper follow-up care. Advances in cancer care are also bringing about more effective treatments with fewer adverse effects.

The following list describes some of the long-term and late effects associated with standard lung cancer treatments. Keep in mind that some patients do not experience any long-term problems as a result of their treatment, although it is more common that you will have some lingering effects. If you experience chronic long-term pain as a result of your cancer treatment, you should not learn to live with it. Ask your doctor for a referral to a pain clinic.

- *Surgery.* Depending on the extent of your surgery, you will likely have reduced lung function, creating physical limitations. This function might improve over time as your remaining lung tissue expands, but it might never return to presurgery capacity. You could also have numbness and nerve pain at and around the surgical site. Other reported late effects include muscle and bone pain and heartburn/reflux, resulting from shifts in your musculoskeletal system and esophagus following lung surgery.

- *Chemotherapy.* Peripheral neuropathy is a common long-term effect of cisplatin or Taxol chemotherapy (see Question 74). Hearing loss or ringing in the ears is experienced occasionally with high doses of cisplatin. Permanent damage to fertility is possible. Some patients also report a reduction in mental function (fuzzy thinking and problems with memory) that is frequently referred to as chemo brain. It is not uncommon for patients to experience fatigue that persists long after chemotherapy has ended. Some drugs can cause permanent kidney (cisplatin) and heart (doxorubicin) damage as well as increase the risk of a second malignancy, such as leukemia. Fortunately, these are extremely rare.

- *Radiation Therapy.* Radiation to the chest can cause permanent scarring in the lungs (**radiation fibrosis**), thereby creating significant long-term breathing problems for some patients. In rare cases, patients can also experience damage to the heart or spine, or

Radiation fibrosis

Scarring of the lungs caused by radiation treatment.

scarring of the esophagus, causing problems swallowing. These serious effects are becoming even less common as advances in technology enable far greater precision in delivering radiation to lung tumors while sparing healthy tissue.

Coping with Symptoms of Lung Cancer

Can my shortness of breath be controlled?

What can I do to relieve my pain?

Am I at risk for a blood clot?
What is a pulmonary embolism?

More . . .

79. Can my shortness of breath be controlled?

There are many causes of shortness of breath, and how to manage it will depend upon the cause. For example, if the shortness of breath is due to a pleural or pericardial effusion, the fluid can be removed to restore breathing capacity (see Question 83). Shortness of breath caused by emphysema or COPD can be managed with inhalers and antibiotics, and pneumonia with antibiotics.

There are several ways to relieve shortness of breath if it is due to the tumor blocking an airway. Radiation is often used to reduce the tumor, thereby relieving the obstruction or blockage. If the patient has already had maximal radiation, a **stent** can sometimes be placed. A stent is a device that looks similar to a hollow tube, which is inserted via bronchoscopy into the airway that is being blocked or crushed by the tumor. Other ways of relieving the obstruction include **brachytherapy**. Brachytherapy is a method of delivering a seed of a radioactive agent into the tumor that is blocking the airway.

Sometimes shortness of breath cannot be controlled using these methods. In these cases, the patient's shortness of breath symptoms can be managed with:

- *Oxygen.* Portable oxygen carriers are available to allow patients to be mobile.
- *Medications, particularly morphine.* Morphine reduces the uncomfortable sensation of breathlessness, so, although a person's body is not getting enough oxygen, the brain does not interpret it this way. Morphine can be given in a number of ways (see Question 81).

Stent

A hollow tube that can be inserted via bronchoscopy into the airway to prevent it from being blocked or crushed by the tumor.

Brachytherapy

Internal radiation therapy that involves placing seeds of radioactive material near or in the tumor.

- *An anti-anxiety medication,* such as lorazepam (Ativan), will also help to relieve your feelings of breathlessness.

80. Could I be depressed?

Depression is a common condition in lung cancer patients. Although patients who have a history of depression are most susceptible, many people who have never before experienced psychiatric problems could develop depression following a lung cancer diagnosis. Even though it is normal and natural to feel sad and down about the diagnosis, sometimes the feelings of sadness become so overwhelming that they take on a life of their own and become a problem in and of themselves. Patients can become so discouraged, hopeless, or full of despair that they are unable to enjoy their family or the little things in life. If you find yourself sitting at home all the time, no longer interested in your usual activities or in getting out of the house, withdrawing from your family, spending all your time in bed, and so on, you could be depressed. The good news is that most depression is treatable—and with medications that are usually well tolerated with minimal side effects. The bad news is that it frequently goes undiagnosed.

Depression is a common condition in lung cancer patients.

Several factors complicate the process of diagnosing depression in cancer patients. For example, many of the symptoms of depression (such as changes in eating and sleeping habits) are also symptoms associated with cancer and its treatment. Also, patients often do not openly share emotional symptoms—a major component of the depression diagnosis—with their doctors. If you think you might be depressed, it is very important that you discuss this possibility with your doctor. If your doctor does diagnose depression, he or she can treat you or refer you to a psychiatrist for further evaluation and treatment. Most frequently, cancer patients have reactive depression. Reactive depression is of limited duration and can be helped with counseling. Major depression is more severe and long lasting, and treatment most often includes medication, such as antidepressants. When depression is treated effectively, patients experience relief from distressing symptoms and are better able to cope with their cancer and the demands of cancer treatment. Recognizing the signs of depression early will help to quickly diagnose and successfully treat it.

Sometimes patients are unwilling to undergo treatment for depression, thinking that it represents a sign of weakness and that they should be able to control their feelings. Nothing could be further from the truth. When you are hungry, you cannot trick your mind into thinking you are not. When you have to go to the bathroom, you cannot trick your mind into thinking you do not. If you are depressed, why would you be able to trick your mind into thinking that you are not?

81. What can I do to relieve my pain?

First and most importantly, talk to your doctor. He or she cannot know you are in pain unless you speak up. Advocate for yourself. If one medication is not effective in relieving your pain, or is causing a lot of side effects, tell your doctor. Do not wait until your next appointment—give the office a call. If they do not call back within a reasonable period of time, call again. You deserve to have relief from pain, and your doctor and nurse would agree with you if you let them know.

Everyone feels pain differently. Your doctor and nurse will often ask you to rate the pain on a scale of 1 to 10, with 0 being no pain and 10 being very severe pain. Some patients agonize over this question, struggling with the difference between a four and a five, and they should not. There is no wrong or right answer, and your nurse or doctor will not quiz you regarding fine differences. This pain scale is simply a general way to determine whether your pain is getting better or worse.

There are many medications for pain. Typically, physicians manage mild pain with non-opioid medications, such as acetaminophen (Tylenol) or nonsteroidal anti-inflammatory drugs (NSAIDs), such as Motrin or Advil. Some type of opioid is usually required for moderate pain. Commonly used preparations include combinations of acetaminophen or NSAIDs with oxycodone or hydrocodone (e.g., Percoset, Vicodan, Norco, and Lortab), administered every 6 hours. Severe pain might require morphine or hydromorphine. Sometimes patients with severe pain might need to be hospitalized for intravenous morphine to quickly control the pain and to determine how much oral morphine they will need as an outpatient.

There are two major types of pain pills—short-acting and long-acting. Short-acting pills typically last about 6 hours and are generally used for pain that is mild, occurs occasionally, or comes and goes. Long-acting pain pills build up to a low but steady level in the blood. They could take a day or 2 to build up to an effective level so don't expect them to work right away. Short-acting pills are used to treat the pain you have at the time; long-acting pain pills are used to prevent it from occurring (or if it does occur, reduce its intensity).

Short-acting pain pills are taken on an as-needed basis. Since long-acting pain pills take awhile to build up in the bloodstream, they must be taken on a very regular basis, whether you are having pain or not.

Many patients feel they shouldn't have to take pain pills. Not so! You will do much better in the long run if you conserve your strength to fight the cancer instead of the pain. Remember—you don't get brownie points for putting up with pain.

Unfortunately, misconceptions about pain medications can sometimes prevent patients from taking these drugs or even talking to their doctor about pain relief. Some common misconceptions include:

- I'm afraid of getting addicted to morphine.

  Don't be. Numerous studies have shown that cancer patients in pain do not get mentally addicted to these drugs. They do not exhibit drug-seeking behavior and are able to be weaned off the medications without difficulty once the cause of the pain is controlled.

- I want to save morphine for when I really need it.

  Don't. Numerous studies have also shown that patients do not become tolerant to these drugs—that is, they do not find themselves requiring more and more pain medications for the same level of pain.

- OK, but I'll still try to get away with taking as few pills as possible.

  Don't. These pain medications are much, much better at preventing pain than taking it away once it starts. These pain medications are designed to be taken on a regular basis, whether you are having pain at that time or not.

- Won't morphine make me woozy and lightheaded?

  It might, but these are side effects that usually go away with repeated treatments. If you have this problem, try starting at a lower dose and slowly working your way up to allow your body to get used to it. If this doesn't work, tell your doctor, and he or she will try a different preparation. Although it varies a lot, some people have more of one kind of side effect on one type of pill than they do with another.

- I'm afraid to take morphine because codeine makes me so constipated.

  This is one of the major problems with these drugs. It is extremely important to try to prevent the constipation—it is much harder to correct constipation after it has already occurred. Talk to your nurse or doctor about the various types of medications recommended to prevent constipation. Typically, most patients start by taking a laxative or stool softener at the same time that they take their pain medications. If you become constipated, try adding milk of magnesia. If that does not work, ask your doctor about taking the same type of medications that are used in preparation for a colonoscopy, such as sorbitol, Go-Lytly, or magnesium citrate.

When using these medications, it is important to know that this is an area where the art of medicine comes in. Everyone is different, so play around with the timing, amount, and combinations of these medications until you have a combination that works for you.

- *What are other side effects of codeine and morphine?*

  Another possible side effect is nausea. Like constipation, if it cannot be managed with medications, ask your doctor to switch you to another type of preparation. Itching is a relatively rare side effect that can also usually be managed with medication.

- *What is the difference between codeine and morphine?*

  Codeine, morphine, oxycodone, hydrocodone, etc., all fit into a class of very similar drugs called opioids. The codeine derivatives—codeine, oxycodone, hydrocodone—tend to be less potent than morphine or its derivatives (hydromorphine, Dilaudid), which simply means that you have to take more of them to get the same effect. They all have the same side effects, though.

- *What is the maximum dose of morphine someone can take?*

  The short answer is, "There is no one maximal dose—it depends on the individual." The side effect that eventually limits the amount of these medications one can take is **respiratory depression**—slowing of breathing. However, most people are able to tolerate very high doses of opioids as long as the dose is increased gradually. A dose that would have very severe side effects in a person who has never taken these drugs might not faze a person who has been on them a while. So, even though patients do not become immune to the pain-killing properties of these medications, with time, they often become tolerant of the side effects.

- *I hate taking pills, period.*

  That is understandable; however, this is a time when the benefits could be far greater than any risks or concerns you might have about a pill. If you have

Respiratory depression

Slowing of breathing.

difficulty swallowing pills, you can ask your doctor about a fentanyl patch. This is a small piece of a plastic-like tape that contains a medication called fentanyl (or Duragesic). This medication gets absorbed through the skin over a 72-hour period of time so the patch needs to be changed about once every 3 days.

- *What is the difference between oxycodone and OxyContin?*

Oxycodone is a derivative of codeine—its effects usually last about 6 hours. OxyContin is a brand name for a long-acting preparation of oxycodone. There are a number of long-acting pain preparations, including OxyContin, MS Contin, Oromorph, among others. All of these medications are coated with a special substance that allows the medication to be slowly absorbed over many hours. The advantage of these medications is that they can greatly reduce the number and frequency of short-acting pain pills one has to take.

For these medications to work well, they have to be taken on a regular schedule. Because they get slowly absorbed, it could take several days for them to start to work. In the meantime, you can continue to take your short-acting pain pills. Indeed, many people have to take a short-acting pain pill occasionally for breakthrough pain.

Because they take longer to work, you might not feel any effects from these medications for a day or 2. Therefore, it is important to take these medications whether you are having pain or not. Like their short-acting counterparts, the long-acting preparations are better at preventing pain than at relieving it, and because they take so long to work, you do not want to suffer tomorrow for not having taken one today. One way of looking at this is that the pill you take today will not be felt until tomorrow.

- *I'm afraid to take these medications, especially OxyContin, after all the stuff I've read about in the newspapers.*

  Don't be. Opioids, when taken for the appropriate reasons by careful individuals, are not harmful or addicting and are true miracle drugs for relieving pain. They only become problematic or addicting when used inappropriately by people who are not in pain.

  OxyContin in particular has been in the press lately. OxyContin is oxycodone (the same medication found in Percoset or Roxicet), but it is somewhat more concentrated. It comes in a preparation that allows the drug to be released slowly over 8 to 12 hours. Some addicts are breaking the pills open and then taking the amount of opioid that is intended to be used over 12 hours all at once. When used appropriately, OxyContin can be very helpful for lung cancer patients.

- *I've tried all these medications. They don't seem to work, and I have too many side effects. I'm afraid nothing more can be done.*

  Not so. Many times pain medication can be much more effectively controlled if it is given continuously through an IV pump. This small device, about the size of a cassette tape recorder, can be easily carried around with you, allowing you to live at home and perform your usual activities.

  If your doctor is not able to effectively manage your pain, ask for a referral to a pain specialist or

If your doctor is not able to effectively manage your pain, ask for a referral to a pain specialist or a palliative care doctor.

a palliative care doctor. They are experts in dealing with the various medications. In addition, they could know whether an injection or nerve block might be helpful.

82. Am I at risk for a blood clot? What is a pulmonary embolism?

A blood clot that occurs in a deep-lying vein in the leg or pelvis is known as a **deep vein thrombosis (DVT)**. If the blood clot breaks off and travels up through the heart and into the lungs, it is called a **pulmonary embolism (PE)**. A pulmonary embolism is a potentially serious condition, because if it is a large blood clot, it can block off a blood vessel going to the lung and cause significant problems with breathing or even death.

Lots of things can cause DVT, particularly in the elderly, including poor circulation, sitting for long periods of time, or being bedridden following surgery. Cancer patients have a higher tendency to get blood clots, probably because some tumors make substances that make the blood more susceptible to clotting. (Clotting is a paraneoplastic syndrome—see Question 9.)

To prevent DVT from happening, your doctor might put you on an anticoagulant (anti-clotting drug), such as coumadin (Warfarin) or heparin. Contrary to popular opinion, these drugs do not cause the blood clot to dissolve. Instead, they prevent the blood clot from becoming even bigger, allowing it to shrivel up and become glued to the wall of the vessel. Although coumadin can work well in some cancer patients, in others it does not. Those patients often need to be treated with heparin. Heparin can be administered in several ways. Until recently, patients were often admitted for intravenous

Deep vein thrombosis (DVT)

A blood clot occurring in a deep-lying vein in the leg or pelvis.

Pulmonary embolism (PE)

A blood clot that travels to the lungs causing full or partial blockage of one or both pulmonary arteries.

Please note that the commonly used phrase, thinning the blood is not quite accurate.

heparin. More recently, low molecular-weight heparin (such as Lovanox) has become available, which can be administered once or twice per day as an injection just under the skin. Please note that the commonly used phrase, thinning the blood is not quite accurate. These medications do not make the blood thinner. They make the blood less likely to clot, allowing the body to take care of the clot as previously described.

83. What are pleural or pericardial effusions, and how are they managed?

A pleural effusion is a collection of fluid between the outside of the lung and the chest wall (the **pleural space**). The lung is covered with a thin membrane called the **visceral pleura**, and the inside of the chest wall is covered with a thin membrane called the **parietal pleura**. Normally, the outside of the lung is touching the chest wall, and the space between the visceral and parietal pleura is virtually non-existent. However, if there are tumor cells on either the visceral pleura, or the parietal pleura, they can become irritated and cause fluid formation.

Pleural space

The area between the outside of the lung and the inside of the chest wall.

Visceral pleura

A membrane surrounding the lung.

Parietal pleura

A membrane lining the chest wall.

Other conditions besides cancer can cause fluid accumulation in the pleural space, including congestive heart failure or pneumonia. To prove that the pleural effusion is indeed due to cancer, your doctor will sample some of the fluid so it can be examined under a microscope by the pathologist. This is typically done as an outpatient procedure by numbing the skin with a topical anesthetic and then inserting a small needle into the chest and draining out some of the fluid.

One of the reasons pleural effusion is significant for lung cancer patients (in addition to the breathing problem it can cause) is that it exists in a free-flowing space. For example, when you stand up, the fluid settles to the bottom of the lung. When you lie on your side, it flows to the side and layers out along the side. If you were to stand on your head, it would flow to the top of the lung. As it flows, it can spread any cancer cells that might be floating within it, thus seeding other areas of either the visceral or parietal pleura. Because the fluid spreads the cancer cells around so extensively, local therapy, such as surgery and radiation, is usually not possible.

In most people, accumulation of some fluid in this area is not a problem. Some people, however, can experience shortness of breath, particularly if the pleural effusion is quite large. When it gets large, patients could also experience an uncomfortable sensation of fullness or discomfort in the chest, as well as a cough.

The pleural effusion can be removed in an outpatient procedure called a **thoracentesis** (see **Figure 3**). In this procedure, a needle is inserted in the back between two ribs. It is attached to a tube that drains the fluid into a bottle or bag. The procedure is relatively painless. The skin is numbed with lidocaine before the needle is inserted, so you will feel the needle to numb the area. After that, most patients do not feel anything, with the possible exception of a cough or vague discomfort if a lot of fluid is removed. These effects are due to the lung re-expanding.

If the fluid keeps reaccumulating, your doctor might recommend a procedure called **pleurodesis**. Although there are several ways of doing this, the procedures are all based upon the principle of draining the lung very, very dry and then inserting some medication into the space where the fluid once was between the chest wall

Thoracentesis

A procedure that uses a needle to remove fluid from the space between the lung and the chest wall.

Pleurodesis

A procedure to prevent recurrence of pleural effusion by draining the fluid and inserting medication into the pleural space.

and lung. This medication is supposed to irritate the covering of the lung and the inside of the chest wall, which in turn is supposed to cause scar tissue (or fibrosis) to form between the two, thus serving as a type of glue to keep the surfaces stuck together. There are a number of different ways of doing this; the size of chest tube, the choice of medication, and whether the tube is inserted in the operating room or at the bedside will vary depending on local practices.

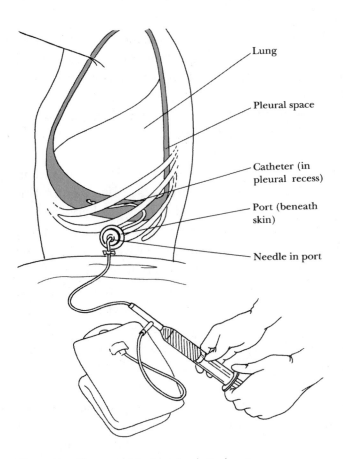

Figure 3   Thoracentesis via an implanted port.

Reprinted from Yarbro CH, Frogge MH, Goodman M, and Groenwald SL. *Cancer Nursing: Principles and Practice*, Sixth Edition. Sudbury, MA: Jones and Bartlett Publishers, LLC, 2005.

Regardless of exactly how the procedure is done, several points should be kept in mind. First, the procedure doesn't always work. This could be because it is impossible to get the pleural space dry enough, or because sometimes the lung will not re-expand. In addition, getting the pleural space as dry as possible often involves between 5–10 days in the hospital, usually with a chest tube inserted. For these reasons, most oncologists do not recommend pleurodesis unless it becomes clear that a patient is going to need repeated thoracentesis.

Sometimes, if a pleurodesis does not work, or if a patient chooses not to undergo the procedure, the surgeon can insert a small, semi-permanent tube called a **Pleurex catheter** into the pleural space that drains to the outside (Figure 3). Fluid can then be drained periodically as it accumulates. Once in place, the tube is painless and cannot be seen under clothing.

Pleurex catheter

Provides symptomatic relief of dyspnea related to recurrent pleural effusions.

Just as the lungs are covered with a thin membrane called the visceral pleura, the heart is covered with a thin membrane called the **pericardium**. A **pericardial effusion** is fluid that accumulates between the heart and the pericardium. Sometimes, this fluid can hinder the heart from beating effectively, and it too might need to be drained in a manner similar to the pleural fluid.

Pericardium

A double-layered serous membrane that surrounds the heart.

Pericardial effusion

Accumulation of fluid inside the sac (pericardium) that surrounds the heart.

84. Is my cough something I should worry about?

Cough is a common symptom that can be due to a number of causes, including lung cancer, infection, smoking, and asthma, among others. If you have a persistent cough, you should tell your doctor. Be prepared to tell him or her how long you have had your cough,

If at any time you cough up blood or see blood in your sputum (the mucus and other material that you cough up from your lungs), you should call your doctor's office immediately.

when and how often your cough occurs, whether your cough produces mucus (and if it does, what color the mucus is), and whether your cough is associated with shortness of breath, wheezing, or fevers. In the majority of cases, your doctor will be able to diagnose and treat your cough effectively with therapy specific for its cause. Persistent coughs can range from a minor annoyance to a major source of fatigue and discomfort for lung cancer patients. Because effective treatment is available for most coughs, and because cough could be a symptom of a serious condition, it makes sense to seek medical attention for a persistent cough. If at any time you cough up blood or see blood in your sputum (the mucus and other material that you cough up from your lungs), you should call your doctor's office immediately.

Living with Lung Cancer

How should I change my diet following a lung cancer diagnosis? Should I take dietary supplements? Can diet affect my survival from lung cancer?

If I smoke, is there any reason to quit? How can I quit smoking while dealing with the stress of lung cancer?

Should I be exercising?

More . . .

85. How should I change my diet following a lung cancer diagnosis? Should I take dietary supplements? Can diet affect my survival from lung cancer?

Many patients wonder whether changing their diet will improve their outcome. Frequently, patients will hear from friends and family that certain diets or foods will make a critical difference in their survival. You might hear, "Drink tons of green tea; it will cure your disease," or "Stay away from sugar; it will feed your tumor." Although some studies have shown that people who consume diets high in fruits and vegetables have a lower risk of developing lung cancer, there is no conclusive evidence that changing your diet after you have been diagnosed with cancer can affect long-term survival.

Although some studies have shown that people who consume diets high in fruits and vegetables have a lower risk of developing lung cancer, there is no conclusive evidence that changing your diet after you have been diagnosed with cancer can affect long-term survival.

This does not mean there is no reason to pay attention to your diet. Eating a healthy diet is good for you and can certainly be beneficial when you are fighting a life-threatening disease. Eating affects how you feel, your energy level, and your overall health. The American Cancer Society's nutrition recommendations include: 1) Eat five or more servings of fruits and vegetables each day; 2) choose whole grains over processed (refined) grains and sugars; 3) limit consumption of red meats, particularly those that are high in fat and are processed; and 4) limit consumption of alcoholic beverages, if you drink at all. Of course, if you are suffering from cancer or treatment-induced weight loss, then you have special dietary needs and your doctor will advise you on what you can do to gain weight, or you can ask your doctor to refer you to a dietician or nutritionist.

There is also no definitive evidence that dietary supplementation can affect your lung cancer. If you do choose to take supplements, alert your doctor so that he or she can advise you as to whether the supplements might interfere with your cancer treatments. It is a good idea to take a multivitamin to ensure you are getting your minimum daily requirements of vitamins and minerals necessary for good health.

Most major medical centers have dieticians or nutritionists who specialize in helping patients with cancer. Ask your doctor or nurse.

86. If I smoke, is there any reason to quit? How can I quit smoking while dealing with the stress of lung cancer?

Yes, there are strong and compelling reasons for smokers to quit following a lung cancer diagnosis. The National Cancer Institute has found that cancer patients who continue to smoke could reduce the effectiveness of their treatment and increase the likelihood of a second cancer. There is also reason to believe that continued smoking could worsen the side effects of treatment, put you at increased risk for complications following lung surgery, and decrease your survival time. One study conducted in small cell lung cancer patients found that survival correlated with smoking status. The patients who continued to smoke after their diagnosis had the poorest survival; the patients who quit at diagnosis fared better; and the patients who had quit on average 2.5 years prior to diagnosis survived the longest.

The National Cancer Institute has found that cancer patients who continue to smoke could reduce the effectiveness of their treatment and increase the likelihood of a second cancer.

Consider how the following health benefits of smoking cessation might affect you at this critical time in your life:

- Your circulation will improve.
- Your pulse rate and blood pressure, which are abnormally high while smoking, will return to normal.
- Your sense of taste and smell will return.
- Your breathing will become easier.
- Your risk of developing infections such as pneumonia (a common cause of death in people with lung cancer) is reduced.
- Your risk of developing other smoking-related diseases, including heart disease and other lung disease, is reduced.

It is never too late to quit. Even following your lung cancer diagnosis, smoking cessation will have a positive impact on your health, your quality of life and, possibly, your survival.

Your challenge is to motivate yourself to quit smoking during an extremely stressful time in your life. For some people this is easy—just hearing the words lung cancer is sufficient motivation. For others, the quitting process becomes even more difficult because smoking relieves the anxiety that comes with having lung cancer. Although quitting smoking is hard work (nicotine is very addicting) there are proven methods available to help you. The Surgeon General recommends **nicotine replacement therapy** (in patch, gum, inhaler, and nasal spray forms) and the antidepressant bupropion SR (Zyban) as treatments that increase long-term quit rates. The effectiveness of these drugs is further increased with counseling, including behavior modification therapy, problem-solving or skills training, and social support.

Nicotine replacement therapy

Smoking cessation method that uses nicotine substitutes in various forms, including a patch, gum, inhaler, or nasal spray.

The more intense the counseling, the more likely you are to quit.

Your doctor can help you to find the combination of cessation methods that will work best for you and advise you on smoking cessation programs that are available in your community. Remember that you could have to make several attempts before you succeed—don't get discouraged. Keep trying and don't try to go it alone—seek support when you need it. For information on organizations, programs, and Internet resources to help you stop smoking, see the Appendix.

Not everyone who smokes and is diagnosed with lung cancer is able to quit smoking. Although there are definite health benefits, there are also understandable reasons why it is not possible for some patients with advanced lung cancer to quit. Scientists are learning that addiction to nicotine in some patients is due to chemical imbalances in the brain, making some patients more addicted than others. In those cases, it is important for the patient and the patient's family to let go of any guilt or anger over smoking. Conflict over smoking only serves to add additional stress on top of an already stressful existence. If you or your family cannot come to terms with your continued smoking, you should seek professional counseling to resolve this divisive issue.

If you or your family cannot come to terms with your continued smoking, you should seek professional counseling to resolve this divisive issue.

87. Should I be exercising?

Exercise can improve both your physical and mental health. It is no different when you have lung cancer. The general benefits credited to exercise—increased strength and energy, elevated mood—are even more desirable when you are battling cancer. The problem is that both your cancer and its treatment make exercise more difficult. However, studies in breast cancer patients have demonstrated that a 20- to 30-minute walking program (five to six times per week) during chemotherapy or radiation therapy helps to decrease levels of fatigue and emotional distress and increase sleep quality, physical functioning, and quality of life. In some cases, exercise can provide both relief and distraction. So there are compelling reasons to get out of your chair and walk—even if it's just a few more steps than yesterday.

A useful exercise for lung cancer patients to learn is called abdominal breathing. Abdominal breathing can help to expand your lungs and increase the flow of oxygen. This is especially desirable for patients who have had surgery to remove a portion of their lung(s). Pulmonary therapists can teach you abdominal breathing and provide additional exercises to maximize your breathing capacity. Physical therapists can show you exercises to increase your upper body strength and range of motion. These exercises are not just for rehabilitation; they can help you with the long-term physical changes that result from surgery. If your surgeon has not given you a referral to a physical therapist, ask for one.

88. What should I know about stress and the immune system? How does stress affect my survival and my ability to cope with my disease? Can complementary therapies help to reduce my stress?

A lung cancer diagnosis brings a pile of additional stress into your life: the stress of knowing you have a life-threatening disease; the stress of deciding what treatment to pursue; the stress of the treatment itself; the stress brought on by the impact of your cancer on the lives of your family and on your daily routine; the stress of explaining your lung cancer to your family and friends (and of dealing with their reactions); the stress of how your lung cancer affects your ability to work and your financial situation—the list of cancer-related stressors is seemingly endless. Stress is an undesirable condition that can negatively affect both your physical and mental well-being. Stress can take away your ability to relax, seek peace of mind, and enjoy life. Although there is no evidence that stress will cause your tumor to grow faster or lessen your chances for long-term survival, it makes sense that someone who is highly stressed experiences a reduced quality of life.

The first step in reducing the stress in your life is to identify your stressors—those things causing you stress. Make a list of everything you can think of that brings on anxiety or causes you to feel additional stress, whether cancer-related or not. Take time to think about how you can eliminate these stressors from your life or reduce the negative impact they have on you. Be creative. Delegate whenever possible. Don't be shy about asking for help or backing out of commitments made prior to your diagnosis. People will understand that lung cancer has changed your priorities and that you now have to focus on your health. Don't be tied to activities that have more of a negative effect on your life than a positive effect. You'll be amazed at how much stress you can eliminate when you sit down and take stock of the nonessentials in your life.

Anti-anxiety medications such as Xanax (alprazolam), Valium (diazepam), or Ativan (lorazepam) can also be very helpful in reducing stress.

The ultimate challenge for most patients, however, is the stress brought on by family and financial obligations and by the physical and emotional consequences of having lung cancer. If your ability to cope with these responsibilities interferes with your daily functioning, you should seek professional counseling. Complementary therapies can also help you to manage your stress. If you can find activities that help you to relax and feel less stressed, you will be better able to cope with the challenges that come your way. Complementary therapies used by cancer patients to reduce stress include relaxation and meditation, exercise programs such as yoga and tai chi, hypnotherapy, biofeedback, massage, and art and music therapy. Many cancer centers offer these types of therapies to patients. For further information on complementary therapies, see the Appendix.

89. What about returning to work? I am worried about being able to function at 100%. What are my rights?

Returning to work after time off for cancer treatment can be both physically and psychologically challenging. You might have physical limitations as a result of your treatment, such as breathing problems and fatigue, which make full-time employment difficult. You might also worry about the reactions of your coworkers to your cancer and dread answering their questions about your health. The process of returning to work is different for everyone. Whether yours will be a smooth transition depends on a number of factors: the extent of your physical limitations; your comfort level in sharing information about your cancer with your coworkers; how supportive (and flexible) your employer is about your needs; your attitude toward your work; and the physical and emotional demands of your job.

Before you negotiate the terms of your return to work, it is important that you are aware of your rights and protections under both federal and state law. The Americans with Disabilities Act (ADA) prohibits discrimination by both public and private employers against qualified workers with disabilities or histories of disabilities. The Federal Rehabilitation Act of 1973 ensures that federal employers or companies receiving federal funds cannot discriminate against cancer survivors (among others) in hiring practices, promotions, transfers, and layoffs. You could have additional employment protections depending upon the laws in your state.

Planning for your return to work can make a difference: know your rights, consider how you will respond to questions from coworkers, and think ahead about what accommodations you might require on a short- or long-term basis so that you will be prepared to discuss your options with your employer. See the Appendix for resources that can assist you in determining your employment rights as a cancer survivor, provide information on how to ease your transition back to work, and direct you to resources you can turn to in the event that you suffer workplace discrimination.

90. What happens when my treatment ends? Why don't I feel happy—or at least relieved?

If your treatment has been successful, and there is no evidence of your lung cancer, you have reason to celebrate. Your hopes for long-term survival, and for a normal life with your friends and family, are closer to becoming a reality. Yet, while you might feel happy on one level, you could also feel anxious on another. This is not unusual. With lung cancer, the fear of recurrence is always there. Active treatment might have given you a sense of security; however, now that your treatment has stopped, your level of anxiety could have increased. You might feel somewhat abandoned—most likely you have become used to frequent office or hospital visits, and have developed close relationships with your doctors, nurses, and the receptionists, and now you are not going to see them for a while. You could also be coping with treatment-related side effects—breathing issues, fatigue, peripheral neuropathy—that interfere with daily life. Your support system might disappear when your treatment ends. Family and friends could hear your good news and stop inquiring after you—the cards, emails, phone calls, and visits that had uplifted you in the past could become less frequent or stop entirely. This is a time of transition. It is not surprising that many lung cancer survivors find it difficult to carry on with their lives after finishing treatment.

A lung cancer support group could be helpful to you at this time. Here, you might find other lung cancer survivors who are facing similar circumstances. You will also be able to reach out to newly diagnosed patients. This effort to help others can make you feel good about yourself and remind you about how far you have come. Advocacy organizations can also be a great resource and provide an opportunity for you to get involved and make a difference for this disease. If your anxiety causes you to feel depressed or interferes with your functioning, you should talk to your doctor and ask whether counseling or medication might help to lessen your distress.

This might be a good time to see a therapist for ideas about how to cope better. You should also let your family and friends know that you still need their support even though you are no longer in treatment. They might assume everything is fine unless you take the time to explain your ongoing needs.

The most important thing you can do during this time is to be vigilant about your follow-up care. Although follow-up care for lung cancer varies among doctors, you should be aware of and comfortable with your doctor's recommendations for office visits, blood tests, and scans. If you are worried about recurrence, ask your doctor if there are any chemoprevention trials that might be appropriate for you (see Questions 59 and 97). In addition to your lung cancer-related concerns, you should discuss well care with your doctor. It is important that you take good care of your health (good nutrition, exercise) so that you can be strong in your survival.

The most important thing you can do during this time is to be vigilant about your follow-up care.

What will be most effective for resolving your emotional distress, and sometimes also your treatment side effects, is the passage of time. As each day passes, you will feel more comfortable with your status as a lung cancer survivor. You will adjust to the emotional, physical, and social changes brought about by your lung cancer experience and find a new equilibrium—a new normal—that will carry you through your life.

91. What about follow-up care? How often should I be seen? What is my doctor looking for?

After you have completed treatment for your lung cancer, it is important that you receive regular follow-up care.

LIVING WITH LUNG CANCER

Your doctor will want to see you to check for recurrence of your lung cancer, to manage any long-term effects from your cancer and its treatment, and to monitor for a second lung cancer or other primary cancer.

The American Society of Clinical Oncologists (ASCO) recommends the following follow-up schedule for asymptomatic (not currently showing symptoms of) lung cancer patients treated with curative intent: every 3 months during the first 2 years; every 6 months during years 3 through 5; and yearly thereafter. More frequent visits are warranted for patients with Stage III disease.

At each follow-up visit, your doctor will order certain blood tests, take a medical history, and perform a physical exam. X-rays and CT scans will be ordered regularly to monitor for recurrence in the lungs. Unfortunately, there are no standard recommendations for the frequency of these imaging studies, and practices among lung specialists vary widely. Although the brain and bone are common sites of metastasis in lung cancer, scans to detect metastatic disease (such as a brain MRI or a bone scan) are usually ordered only if symptoms are present.

The purpose of follow-up care, however, is to detect recurrence or disease at an early stage when it can be treated curatively or, if that is not possible, to begin **palliative treatment** in a timely manner. You will want to ask your doctor what symptoms you should be concerned about and under what circumstances you should report them.

Even though you are at high risk of recurrence during the first few years after your diagnosis, your risk declines

Palliative treatment

Treatment given not with the intent to cure but with the intent to prolong survival and reduce symptoms from the tumor.

as time goes on. You remain at increased risk, however, for a second, totally different primary lung cancer. Watching for a second lung cancer is important because **resection** of second primaries can be successful.

Although your main concern during your follow-up visits will undoubtedly be to make sure that your lung cancer has not recurred or that a second lung cancer has not developed, you should not hesitate to bring up other health issues that impact your quality of life. It is not unusual for patients to experience depression when their treatment stops, and you should discuss this with your doctor if you feel depressed or overly anxious and think you might benefit from counseling. Patients who have undergone chemotherapy, radiation, or surgery might experience long-term side effects that should be discussed on a regular basis so they can be properly addressed. (See Question 78 for discussion of long-term and late effects.) Do not feel that your complaints are too minor to bring up during your follow-up visits. Your quality of life is important and your doctor should work with you to address these concerns.

Resection

Surgical removal.

92. Should I get a flu shot? What about the pneumonia vaccine?

Lung infections can pose a serious and potentially deadly threat to lung cancer patients. Safe and effective vaccines are available for both influenza (the flu) and pneumo-coccal pneumonia, two common lung infections. Note that these vaccines protect against two very specific diseases—influenza and pneumococcal pneumonia—and therefore are not a guarantee you will not contract another respiratory illness, such as the common cold.

Don't wait to ask your doctor about getting vaccinated; it could save your life.

The flu shot is administered yearly, most optimally in October or November. You can get the pneumonia vaccine at any time, and revaccination is recommended after 5 years. Don't wait to ask your doctor about getting vaccinated; it could save your life.

If Treatment Fails

How do I decide if it's time to stop treatment?

What is hospice?

What can I do to prepare for my death?

More . . .

93. How do I decide if it's time to stop treatment?

Deciding when to stop treatment is an extremely difficult and personal decision that no one can make for you. Each person must come to this point on his or her own terms—there is no one way for you to decide. Often decisions to stop treatment come about when the side effects of treatment outweigh any potential benefit. However, this decision is deeply personal and can result from a number of circumstances occurring at the same time. Most importantly, it should be based on your values and beliefs. You might seek counsel from the people who have helped you to make decisions along the way—this could include family members, friends, healthcare providers, spiritual advisors, and others. Family members and friends can provide guidance and support as you struggle with your decision, but you should realize that their counsel will be charged with their own emotions and views. This might create conflict and make the decision more difficult for you. They might not be ready. On the other hand, you could find that the view of your family is in line with yours, thereby making your decision easier. Ultimately, however, it is your decision to make. There is no way to predict how you will come to a decision to stop treatment and how others will react to your decision. What matters most is that you are at peace with the decision you have made.

There is no way to predict how you will come to a decision to stop treatment and how others will react to your decision.

94. What is hospice?

Hospice began as a philosophy for how end-of-life care should be provided. Today, hospice organizations provide palliative care to dying patients, usually in their homes. Hospice patients are cared for by a team that could include doctors, nurses, nursing assistants, social workers, therapists, spiritual advisors, counselors, and hospice volunteers, among others. Although most hospices do not provide 24-hour care, hospices do provide a wide range of support to the terminally ill by addressing their medical, emotional, spiritual, and practical needs as well as by providing support for family members. Typical services include providing equipment and oxygen in the home; nursing assistants to help with bathing; nursing services to administer intravenous pain medications; social worker support; and grief counseling. One of the big advantages of hospice (in addition to providing equipment and medications) is that the hospice nurses act as your doctor's eyes and ears, decreasing the number of trips to the doctor for problems. In addition, they can give IV medications and fluids at home, which is much more convenient.

A primary focus of hospice care is to provide symptom relief, and hospice professionals are particularly expert at pain management. Many patients choose hospice care to ensure that their final days will be as pain-free as possible. Some hospices allow chemotherapy, providing it is given for palliative purposes; most hospices allow radiotherapy for the same reason.

Most often, hospices provide care at home, but some hospices also have in-patient hospice centers or long-term care facilities. The range and amount of hospice services available to you will depend on your local hospice and on your insurance plan. Hospice coverage is provided by Medicare and often also by Medicaid and private insurance providers. For further information on hospice and how to locate hospice services, see the resources listed in the Appendix.

Many hospices state they are for patients with less than 6 months to live, which of course is very scary. However, this is *not* a hard and fast rule—it is merely meant to be a guideline. Also, you can be on hospice and then come off if things get better.

Most hospices like to meet possible patients well in advance, even before they are needed. This allows them to meet the patient and family in a more relaxed setting, so they are not coming into an emergency situation. That way, they get to know you, your particular situation, and can describe the services they offer. Ask your doctor for a referral if you think you might need hospice at some point.

95. What can I do to prepare for my death?

In the middle of agonizing emotions and physical challenges, patients who are dying have important decisions to make. Addressing these end-of-life issues proactively can help terminally ill patients to resolve physical, psychological, and practical challenges in a way that is consistent with personal beliefs. Hopefully this will provide some measure of comfort and peace of mind to both patient and family.

Talk to your doctor about his or her comfort level in handling end-of-life issues. If he or she is not comfortable in handling these issues, or has done so only rarely, you might want to seek a palliative care consultation. A palliative care doctor specializes in the needs of terminally ill patients. You deserve to have symptom management and relief from pain during your final days, and you might want to consider hospice care at this time (see

Question 94). It is critical that you communicate your wishes about your medical care at the end of life to your healthcare providers. **Advance directives** will allow you to prepare for the medical possibilities and assign some-one who can act on your behalf, should you become unable to direct your own medical care (see Question 96). Your views on what quality of life and death with dignity mean to you are appropriate topics to discuss with both your doctors and the person you have desig-nated to act on your behalf (also called a **healthcare proxy**).

Think about your emotional and spiritual needs. Fear or denial of approaching death, or anxiety about the dying process, is common. You might want to find someone with whom you can discuss your feelings about death and dying. This could be your doctor, your reli-gious leader, a family member, or a close friend. Many patients also explore the meaning of their lives and of their cancer experiences during this time. This spiritual journey is important to patients, regardless of their reli-gious background and practice.

Take care of financial affairs including making sure your will is in order. Though it is difficult to deal with these sensitive concerns, it will lessen the burdens on your family after your death.

Attend to unfinished business—settle up emotional accounts. Make amends; say your goodbyes. Spend time with those who mean the most to you.

A palliative care specialist, hospice, your doctor, or a social worker will be able to refer you to end-of-life sup-port resources. By preparing for your eventual death, you will help yourself and your family to cope with the

Advance directives

Legal documents that allow you to prepare for future medical possibilities and to assign some-one to act on your behalf in the event you become unable to direct your own medical care.

Healthcare proxy

A person you have designated to make healthcare deci-sions for you in the event you become incapacitated.

Advance directives will allow you to prepare for the medical pos-sibilities and assign someone who can act on your behalf, should you become unable to direct your own medical care.

dying process. Many terminally ill patients worry that they will be a burden to their families. This is less likely to occur when you have addressed these issues ahead of time. You'll have peace of mind knowing that you have done all you can to spare your family additional stress. You can then concentrate on your quality of life and on sharing time with your loved ones during your final days.

96. What are advance directives?

Advance directives are legal documents that specify your wishes regarding your future medical care. They are used in the event that you become unable to make these decisions yourself. As a patient, you have the right to accept or refuse medical treatment; advance directives protect this right.

You should familiarize yourself with these three types of advance directives:

Do Not Resuscitate (DNR) order

An advance directive stating you do not want doctors to do whatever is necessary to keep you alive in the event of a cardiac or respiratory arrest.

Do Not Resuscitate (DNR) order. Your doctor might (in fact, should) ask you about a DNR order. This can be a very uncomfortable subject to discuss, but it is something everyone should think about, regardless of one's health. Your doctor wants to know whether, in the event of a cardiac or respiratory arrest (e.g., a massive heart attack or if you stop breathing, regardless of the reason), you would want heroic measures performed—that is, whether you would want doctors to do whatever is necessary to keep you alive. These measures could involve shocking your chest, putting in a breathing tube, or putting you on a ventilator (breathing machine) in the intensive care unit. Some considerations to keep in mind before you decide:

- *How strong are you?* Very weak patients rarely recover enough to eventually get off the breathing machine and leave the intensive care unit, even if it was not cancer that caused their heart or lungs to stop.

- *Why did this happen?* If it happened because of a complication of the lung cancer, and if the lung cancer is advanced and unlikely to be controlled, the chances of successfully coming off the ventilator are very remote.

- *How difficult will it be for your family to decide when to stop trying?* (Often thought of as the when-to-pull-the-plug decision.)

There are several reasons why it is very important that you think about this issue and discuss it with your family before you get seriously ill.

- It is much easier to be calm and objective when talking about a hypothetical event.

- Very often, the heart or lungs can stop working suddenly, and there is not time to have a discussion as to whether to try to revive the patient. If a DNR order has not been written, the patient will almost always be coded, and an attempt to resuscitate the patient will be made.

This is the one type of advance directive that does not require your signature—your doctor can write an order on your chart after having discussed it with you. Also, should you decide to be DNR, ask your doctor or nurse about a DNR bracelet. This is a small plastic band, similar to a hospital identification band, worn around the wrist that indicates you do not want to be resuscitated in the event of a cardiac or respiratory arrest. This bracelet will prevent paramedics from trying to resuscitate you should you collapse out in public.

Sometimes patients are reluctant to be made DNR, thinking that it means that no treatment will be given for anything, and that the doctor is giving up on them.

Living will

A document in which you specify which medical treatments you do and do not want to have should you become unable to decide for yourself.

Sometimes patients are reluctant to be made DNR, thinking that it means that no treatment will be given for anything, and that the doctor is giving up on them.

Nothing could be further from the truth. DNR does *not* mean do not treat—the type of treatment you want for your cancer or other conditions, if any, is between you and your doctor. DNR simply means that you will not be put on a breathing machine should you have a heart attack or stop breathing.

Living will. A living will is a document in which you specify which medical treatments you do and do not want to have should you become unable to decide for yourself. Because one cannot anticipate every eventuality, most healthcare providers recommend a medical power of attorney rather than a living will. It is important that you discuss your living will with your doctor. Your doctor can explain any medical and ethical details that you need to know in order to make decisions about end-of-life care. The National Cancer Institute recommends that you consider the following life-sustaining measures when drawing up your living will:

- The use of life-sustaining equipment (dialysis machines, ventilators, and respirators)
- Do not resuscitate (DNR) orders; artificial hydration and nutrition (tube feeding)
- Withholding of food and fluids
- Palliative/comfort care
- Organ and tissue donation

A critical part of the living will process is to discuss your wishes with your family and loved ones. This will allow them to more easily understand and accept your decisions.

Durable power of attorney for health care. A durable power of attorney for health care is also known as a medical power of attorney. This type of advance directive allows you to specify a healthcare proxy—a trusted person such as your spouse or other loved one—to make medical decisions for you should you become unable to do so for yourself. You should share your general and specific views regarding life-sustaining care and end-of-life issues with the person who will be your healthcare proxy, and make sure this person will be able to make your medical decisions for you—even under circumstances in which your wishes might not be known.

Most hospitals, lawyers, and palliative care physicians recommend a durable power of attorney over a living will because a living will can never foresee all possibilities as to what could happen to a person. If you have designated a power of attorney, however, and this person knows you well, he or she probably will know what you would want done regardless of the circumstance.

Sources for additional information on preparing advance directives can be found in the Hospice and End-of-Life Issues section in the Appendix. Copies of signed documents should be given to your doctor and to your healthcare proxy.

You shouldn't worry that by preparing an advance directive; you are giving up on your hope for survival or turning your lung cancer into an automatic death sentence. Ideally, everyone should have advance directives—not just people with serious or life-threatening conditions. By dealing with these difficult end-of-life issues ahead of time, and by discussing them with your family and loved ones, you will have removed a potential source of distress for them and given yourself peace of mind that your wishes will be carried out.

Durable power of attorney for health care

An advance directive that allows you to specify a healthcare proxy to make medical decisions for you should you become unable to do so for yourself.

IF TREATMENT FAILS

Prevention, Screening, and Advocacy

Can lung cancer be prevented?
What is chemoprevention?

Does lung cancer run in families? Is my family at increased risk for lung cancer because I have lung cancer?

Why has there been so little progress in fighting lung cancer? What can I do to help?

More . . .

97. Can lung cancer be prevented? What is chemoprevention?

A key to preventing lung cancer is smoking prevention and cessation. Active smoking is responsible for 85%–90% of all lung cancers, and exposure to secondhand smoke accounts for a significant portion of the remaining cases. But it's incorrect to consider lung cancer as only a smoker's disease. About 15% of people diagnosed with lung cancer have never smoked. In addition, about half of all lung cancers in the United States occur in people who have given up smoking. Although the risk of developing lung cancer goes down with smoking cessation, it never goes away completely. A significant risk remains for 20 years or longer after quitting.

Active smoking is responsible for 85%–90% of all lung cancers, and exposure to secondhand smoke accounts for a significant portion of the remaining cases.

Preventing people from smoking would no doubt result in a vast reduction in the incidence of lung cancer. Tragically, there has been little progress toward reaching this goal. Tobacco companies continue to be effective in marketing their deadly product to teenagers, who are likely to ignore the risks associated with smoking. Messages that promote smoking as a cool behavior are rampant throughout our culture, making a mockery of anti-smoking campaigns. Public health initiatives in smoking prevention have not succeeded—we need more and more effective, school-based prevention programs beginning in preschool. And children and adults who are already smoking deserve better access to resources that will help them quit. Although smoking cessation will reduce the likelihood of getting lung cancer, a smoker's risk will never be equal to that of a non-smoker. The best advice for preventing lung cancer is to never start smoking and to avoid chronic exposure to secondhand smoke. Other environmental hazards, such as exposure to asbestos and radon, are responsible for a small percentage of lung cancer cases. Federal safety regulations are helping to prevent exposure to these and other lung carcinogens in the workplace.

Clinical trials are under way to determine whether lung cancer can be prevented in people who are at high risk for the disease, such as current and former smokers and people with a history of lung cancer. These studies are called chemoprevention trials. They are designed to test whether natural or chemical substances can prevent cancer.

Findings from previous chemoprevention trials involving beta-carotene and alpha-tocopherol (a type of vitamin E) were discouraging. The results in some cases showed that these supplements actually increased the incidence of lung cancer in smokers. As more is learned about lung **carcinogenesis**, scientists continue to test promising chemopreventive agents. If your lung cancer is in remission, you could be a candidate for a chemoprevention trial. Ask your doctor whether this might be a good option for you. Because increased participation will help find ways to prevent lung cancer, you should encourage your family and friends who are current or former smokers to consider chemoprevention trials. For information on locating chemoprevention trials, see the Appendix.

Carcinogenesis
The development of cancer.

98. Is there a screening test for lung cancer? Should my loved ones be screened?

It is important to first understand what a screening test is. A screening test looks at asymptomatic individuals (people without symptoms) with a particular risk factor for a disease in hopes of making an early diagnosis. Making an earlier diagnosis is not enough, however;

for a screening test to be useful, the earlier diagnosis must result in fewer people dying of the disease, or at least living longer. This is different from a diagnostic test, which is done to confirm the presence of a disease in a patient who already has symptoms.

In the past, chest X-rays have been used for lung cancer screening on an informal basis, and there are lung cancer specialists who believe that chest X-rays done in high-risk populations find enough early cancers to justify their use as a screening test. However, most specialists feel that by the time a lung cancer has grown to the point that it can be seen on a chest X-ray, it may have already spread to other parts of the body. Randomized screening trials in the 1970s failed to show that smokers who underwent annual chest X-rays were less likely to die of lung cancer than those who did not. Therefore, the American Cancer Society does not recommend a chest X-ray as a screening tool for lung cancer.

A promising new technology called a low-dose spiral CT scan has been shown to be better at detecting small lung abnormalities (nodules) than X-ray. Low-dose spiral CT is an advanced technology that can generate a three-dimensional image of internal structures in seconds. They are more successful at catching lung nodules (potentially cancerous cells). A recent randomized clinical trial called the National Lung Cancer Screening Trial (NLST) found a 20 percent reduction in deaths from lung cancer among current or former heavy smokers who were screened with low-dose helical CT versus those screened by chest X-ray. The results of this trial are currently being reviewed by the US Preventive Services Task Force and various insurance agencies to determine if it is "cost-effective" to be recommended.

What is the down side to physicians routinely recommending spiral CT screening? Why not just order them on everyone? It turns out that a large percentage of people (in some studies, over 70%) have very small abnormalities on CT scans and, in most cases it is unclear what these abnormalities are. Thus, many people need to be followed with repeat CT scans for years before the radiologist feels comfortable calling abnormalities benign. In addition to the anxiety these tests will produce, there is a small risk associated with exposing people to radiation from repeat CTs if they do not need them. Furthermore, some patients end up having biopsies of what turns out to be benign lesions, and there is some risk and discomfort associated with that as well. For all these reasons, physicians are sometimes reluctant to routinely recommend screening CTs. Currently, most insurance companies are not paying for the screening CT.

Needless to say, this is a rapidly changing field. By the time you read this, it is almost certain that more professional organizations and health agencies will have made recommendations regarding the use of low dose spiral CTs in routine screening for people who are at a high risk for developing lung cancer.

99. Does lung cancer run in families? Is my family at increased risk for lung cancer because I have lung cancer?

Some families do have a high incidence of lung cancer. Scientists are studying these families to determine why certain people are at greater risk for developing this deadly disease. It could be that in some cases, blood relatives with lung cancer share genetic mutations (abnormalities) that make them more susceptible to smoking and other environmental carcinogens. This is probably due to the fact that some people do not metabolize (neutralize and excrete) carcinogens (cancer-causing substances) in cigarette smoke as well as others, and this characteristic can be inherited. Several studies have suggested that women might be more susceptible to developing lung cancer than men, and the difference in metabolizing carcinogens could be one reason why.

Although our present understanding is limited, research into families with lung cancer is shedding light on the complex relationship among the lifestyle, environmental, and genetic factors that make up lung cancer risk.

Currently, there is no genetic test to determine risk for lung cancer. Thus, there is no way to know whether your family (particularly your siblings and children) might be at increased risk because of your lung cancer. As genetic markers for lung cancer risk continue to be identified and characterized, this could change. It makes sense for anyone with a family history of lung cancer to discuss this, and other risk factors, with his or her doctor. There are no recommendations for widespread screening for lung cancer, although a doctor might choose to do this for individuals in certain cases.

Even though there could be trends for increased susceptibility for getting lung cancer that run in families, at this point there have not been any genes known to cause lung cancer which can be inherited and passed down from generation to generation. *EGFR mutations and ALK abnormalities occur only in the cancer cells and therefore cannot be inherited.*

If two or more members of your family have lung cancer, you might be able to participate in a family research study. For more information, contact the Johns Hopkins National Familial Lung Cancer Registry by phone at (410) 614-1910 or visit its website at *www.path.jhu.edu/nfltr.html.*

100. Why has there been so little progress in fighting lung cancer? What can I do to help?

It is frustrating to learn that although lung cancer is the number one cancer killer of men and women in the United States, research is funded at significantly lower levels than the other common cancers. Lung cancer advocates have long argued that this disparity exists because lung cancer is associated with smoking and perceived by the public as a self-inflicted disease. This smoking stigma affects both public support and media coverage of lung cancer. It also affects the willingness of people with lung cancer to stand up and speak out about this deadly disease. Many lung cancer survivors feel guilty about their smoking and fear public scorn if they were to demand more dollars for lung cancer research. And, for many people with lung cancer, the possibility of becoming an advocate is out of the question— the sad fact is that the overwhelming majority of people with lung cancer will not survive their disease. They are too sick to advocate for themselves, and their families are too grief-stricken to spend the emotional energy. In addition, although there are numerous advocacy organizations for breast, colon, and prostate cancers, there are far fewer organizations advocating on behalf of lung cancer patients.

There are countless ways that individuals can help to effect the changes necessary to make strategy for progress a reality. Here are a few places to start.

Familiarize yourself with lung cancer issues. Read everything on lung cancer that you can find. Think about how these issues affect you, and how they affect other lung cancer survivors, as well as people at risk for lung cancer.

Contact a lung cancer advocacy organization such as the National Lung Cancer Partnership. (See the Appendix for contact information.) Let them know you are interested in participating in advocacy activities. Advocacy organizations initiate and coordinate efforts to influence policy and funding for lung cancer research, raise awareness of lung cancer, and increase support services for people with lung cancer.

Support lung cancer research. Breast cancer advocates have been remarkably successful in raising money for research, and many feel that this is one reason why the breast cancer cure rate has gone up. A number of lung cancer advocacy organizations raise money for research—tell your friends and family.

Let your voice be heard. Write to your representatives in Washington and to your local media about lung cancer and lung cancer issues. Volunteer to participate in school anti-smoking programs. Visit local hospitals and advocate for increased information, education, and support services for lung cancer patients. Advocacy organizations can provide guidance and materials for these types of efforts and connect you with other survivors who are interested in effecting change. Remember, there is strength in numbers. Lung cancer advocates are working hard to network with each other and to follow the progress that has come about for breast, prostate, and colon cancers. Our voices are gradually becoming a chorus.

Put a face on lung cancer. You do not have to become a full-time advocate to make a difference in the fight against lung cancer. Each time you identify yourself as a lung cancer survivor, you are putting a face on lung cancer. You are telling the world that people with lung cancer matter and deserve the same respect as people with other forms of cancer. You are bringing others into the lung cancer community. This is a battle we all can win together.

PREVENTION, SCREENING, AND ADVOCACY

Where Can I Find More Information?

Lung Cancer Information

National Lung Cancer Partnership

Website: *www.NationalLungCancerPartnership.org*
Phone: (608) 233-7905
1 Point Place, Suite 200, Madison, WI 53719

The National Lung Cancer Partnership is the only national nonprofit lung cancer organization founded by physicians and researchers with lung cancer survivors and advocates. Its mission is to decrease deaths due to lung cancer and help patients live longer and better through research, awareness, and advocacy.

American Society of Clinical Oncology (ASCO)

Website: *www.asco.org*
Phone: (703) 299-0150
2318 Mill Road, Suite 800, Alexandria, VA 22314

ASCO is a professional organization for cancer doctors. New findings in cancer research are presented each year at its annual conference. Conference abstracts are posted on the ASCO Website.

CancerCare

Website: *www.lungcancer.org*
Phone: (800) 813-HOPE (4673)
275 Seventh Avenue, New York, NY 10001

A national nonprofit organization that provides free, professional support services to anyone affected by lung cancer. Services include counseling, education, financial assistance, and practical help. Information is available in Spanish.

Cancer.net

Website: *www.cancer.net*

Oncologist-approved information for people with cancer; maintained by the American Society for Clinical Oncology (ASCO).

Florida Lung Cancer Partnership
(See National Lung Cancer Partnership)

Website: *www.fllungcancerpartnership.org*
2200 Kings Hwy Building 3L, Suite 196, Punta Gorda, FL 33980

International Association for the Study of Lung Cancer (IASLC)

Website: *www.iaslc.org*
Phone: (855) GO-IASLC (46-42752)
13100 East Colfax Avenue, Unit 10, Aurora, CO 80011

IASLC is a professional organization that promotes research into all aspects of lung cancer and thoracic malignancies and encourages world-wide cancer prevention efforts.

Louisiana Lung Cancer Partnership (See National Lung Cancer Partnership)

Website: *www.lalungcancerpartnership.org*
Phone: (337) 478-4538
P.O. Box 548, Lake Charles, LA 70602

Caring Ambassadors Lung Cancer Program

Website: *www.lungcancercap.org*
Phone: (503) 632-9032
P.O. Box 1748, Oregon City, OR 97045

Through state-of-the-art information, awareness efforts, advocacy, and support, the Caring Ambassadors Lung Cancer Program (CAP Lung Cancer) is firmly committed to bettering the lives of people living with lung cancer and their loved ones.

National Cancer Institute (NCI)

Website: *www.cancer.gov*
Phone: (800)-4CANCER
(NCI's Cancer Information Service)
NCI Public Inquiries Office, 6116 Executive Blvd., Room 3036A, Bethesda, MD 20892

The NCI offers extensive up-to-date online and print information on lung cancer and its treatment, including clinical trials. Information is also available in Spanish.

North Carolina Lung Cancer Partnership
(See National Lung Cancer Partnership)
Website: *www.nclungcancerpartnership.org*
Phone: (919) 784-0410
Email: info@nclungcancerpartnership.org
4000 Blue Ridge Road, Suite 170, Raleigh, NC 27612

Pennsylvania Lung Cancer Partnership
(See National Lung Cancer Partnership)
Website: *www.palungcancerpartnership.org*

Uniting Against Lung Cancer
Website: *www.unitingagainstlungcancer.org*
Phone: (212) 627-5500
27 Union Square West, Suite 304, New York, NY 10003

Uniting Against Lung Cancer (UALC) is dedicated to funding innovative research and raising awareness to find a cure for lung cancer.

Print Publications
Henschke, C., et al. *Lung Cancer: Myths, Facts, Choices—and Hope*. New York: W. W. Norton, 2002.

Johnston, L. Lung Cancer: Making Sense of Diagnosis, Treatment, and Options. Sebastopol, CA: O'Reilly & Associates, 2001.

CURE: Cancer Updates, Research and Education. Quarterly magazine that aims to explain scientific information to cancer patients. Print subscription is free to patients at *www.curetoday.com*.

Caregivers and Home Care
Family Caregiver Alliance
Website: *www.caregiver.org*
Phone: (415) 434-3388; toll-free: (800) 445-8106
785 Market Street, Suite 750, San Francisco, CA 94103

Caregiver resources include an online support group and an information clearinghouse. Information is also available in Spanish.

National Family Caregivers Association

Website: *www.nfcacares.org*

Phone: (301) 942-6430; toll-free: (800) 896-3650

10400 Connecticut Avenue, Suite 500, Kensington, MD 20895-3944

NFCA provides education, information, support, and advocacy services for family caregivers.

CAREGIVERS (Association of Cancer Online Resources)

Website: *www.acor.org* (Enter Caregivers in the search box)

Online discussion group for caregivers of cancer patients.

Guide for Cancer Supporters: Step-by-Step Ways to Help a Relative or Friend Fight Cancer (R.A. Bloch Cancer Foundation)

Website: *www.blochcancer.org*

Print Publications

Houts, PS and Bucher, JA, eds. *Caregiving: A Step-by-Step Resource for Caring for the Person with Cancer at Home.* Atlanta, GA: American Cancer Society, 2000.

Children

Kids Konnected

Website: *www.kidskonnected.org*

Phone: (949) 582-5443; toll-free: (800) 899-2866

26071 Merit Circle, Suite 103, Laguna Hills, CA 92653

Nationwide organization that provides extensive support resources and programs for children who have a parent with cancer.

Print Publications

Harpham, WS. *When a Parent Has Cancer: A Guide to Caring for Your Children*, with companion book *Becky and the Worry Cup: A Children's Book about a Parent's Cancer.* New York: Perennial Currents, 2004.

Clinical Trials Resources

There is no single resource for locating clinical trials for lung cancer. It makes sense to check repeatedly with all of the resources listed below because new trials are continually added. Clinical trials services are also emerging to help match patients to clinical trials. Some of these services can be useful for obtaining information and saving time, but it is important to read the company's privacy statement before using them and know whether the company is being paid for recruiting patients.

NCI Clinical Trials
Website: *www.cancer.gov*
Phone: (800)-4CANCER

The National Cancer Institute (NCI) offers comprehensive information on understanding and finding clinical trials, including access to the NCI/ PDQ Clinical Trials Database.

NIH/NLM Clinical Trials
Website: *www.cancer.gov/clinicaltrials/search*

Clinical trials database service developed by the National Institutes of Health's National Library of Medicine.

Centerwatch Clinical Trials Listing Service
Website: *www.centerwatch.com*

Listing of clinical trials, including trials sponsored by drug companies.

Clinical Trials Resources
Website: *www.lungcanceronline.org*

In addition to linking to the major clinical trials resources listed above, Lungcanceronline.org provides links to NCI-designated cancer centers and hospitals with lung cancer programs that are likely to be conducting clinical trials in lung cancer. These sites can be contacted directly for information on available lung cancer trials. Links to some clinical trials services and directly to drug company trial information can also be found in Lungcanceronline.org's clinical trials section.

NCI Clinical Trials and Insurance Coverage

Website: *www.cancer.gov*

Excellent in-depth guide to clinical trials' insurance issues.

Print Publications

Finn, R. *Cancer Clinical Trials: Experimental Treatments and How They Can Help You.* Sebastopol, CA: O'Reilly & Associates, 1999.

Mulay, M. *Making the Decision: A Cancer Patient's Guide to Clinical Trials.* Sudbury, MA: Jones and Bartlett Publishers, LLC, 2002.

Complementary and Alternative Medicine (CAM)

American Academy of Medical Acupuncture

Website: *www.medicalacupuncture.org*
Phone: (310) 364-0193
1970 E. Grand Ave, Suite 330, El Segundo, California 90245

Professional site with articles on acupuncture, a list of frequently asked questions, and acupuncturist locator.

National Center for Complementary and Alternative Medicine (NCCAM)

Website: *www.nccam.nih.gov*

Offers information on complementary and alternative medicine therapies, including NCI/PDQ expert-reviewed fact sheets on individual therapies and dietary supplements.

NCI Office of Cancer Complementary and Alternative Medicine (OCCAM)

Website: *www.cancer.gov*

Information clearinghouse supporting the NCI's CAM activities.

Print Publications

American Cancer Society. *American Cancer Society's Guide to Complementary and Alternative Cancer Methods*. Atlanta, GA: American Cancer Society, 2000.

Kaptchuk, TJ. *The Web That Has No Weaver: Understanding Chinese Medicine*. New York: McGraw-Hill, 2000.

Diet and Nutrition

American Institute for Cancer Research

Website: *www.aicr.org*
Phone: (202) 328-7744; toll-free: (800) 843-8114
1759 R Street, NW, Washington, DC 20009

Supports research on diet and nutrition in the prevention and treatment of cancer. Provides information to cancer patients on nutrition and cancer, including a compilation of healthy recipes. Maintains a nutrition hotline for questions relating to nutrition and health.

Nutrition (American Cancer Society)

Website: *www.cancer.org* (Enter Nutrition in the search box.)

Nutrition resources include ACS guidelines on nutrition, dietary supplement information, nutrition message boards, and tips on low-fat cooking and choosing healthy ingredients.

Drugs/Medications

MedlinePlus: Drug Information

Website: *www.medlineplus.gov* (Click on Drugs & Supplements.)

Database with information on thousands of prescription and over-the-counter medications. Maintained by the National Library of Medicine.

Print Publications

Wilkes, G. *Consumers Guide to Cancer Drugs*. Sudbury, MA: Jones and Bartlett Publishers, LLC, 2003.

Employment, Insurance, Financial, and Legal Resources

Americans with Disabilities Act (U.S. Department of Justice)

Website: *www.ada.gov*

Provides information and technical assistance related to the ADA.

America's Health Insurance Plans (AHIP)

Website: *www.ahip.org*

Provides insurance guides for consumers. Topics include health insurance, managed care, disability income, and long-term care.

Cancer Legal Resource Center

Website: *www.lls.edu/academics*
Phone: (213) 736-1000; toll-free: (866) THE-CLRC
919 S. Albany Street, Los Angeles, CA 90015

A joint program of the Disability Rights Legal Center and Loyola Law School. Provides free information and resources on cancer-related legal issues to survivors, caregivers, healthcare professionals, employers, and others coping with cancer.

Centers for Medicare and Medicaid Services (CMS) (Formerly the Health Care Financing Administration [HCFA])

Website: *www.cms.hhs.gov*

The CMS is a federal agency within the U.S. Department of Health and Human Services that oversees administration of:

Medicare

Website: *www.medicare.gov*
Phone: (800) MEDICARE

Federal health insurance program for people 65 years or older and some disabled people under 65 years.

Medicaid

Website: *www.medicaid.gov*

Federal and state health assistance program for certain low-income people.

Health Insurance Portability and Accountability Act (HIPAA)
Website: *www.cms.hhs.gov*

Insurance reform that might lower your chance of losing existing coverage, ease your ability to switch health plans and/or help you buy coverage on your own if you lose your employer's plan and have no other coverage available.

Family and Medical Leave Act (FMLA)
Website: *www.dol.gov* (Enter FMLA in the search box.)

U.S. Department of Labor Website, providing information about the Family and Medical Leave Act (FMLA).

Hill-Burton Program
(Health Resources and Services Administration)
Website: *www.hrsa.gov* (Enter Hill-Burton Program in the search box.)
Phone: (800) 638-0742; in Maryland: (800) 492-0359

Facilities that receive Hill-Burton funds from the government are required by law to provide free services to some people who cannot afford to pay. Information on Hill-Burton eligibility and facilities locations is available via phone or Internet.

Patient Advocate Foundation
Website: *www.patientadvocate.org*
Phone: (800) 532-5274
421 Butler Farm Road, Hampton, VA 23666

Nonprofit organization helps patients to resolve insurance, debt, and job discrimination matters relative to their cancer diagnosis through case managers, doctors, and attorneys.

Social Security Administration (SSA)
Website: *www.ssa.gov*
Phone: (800) 772-1213

Oversees two programs that pay benefits to people with disabilities:
- Social Security Disability Insurance—pays benefits to you and certain members of your family if you have worked long enough and paid Social Security taxes.
- Supplemental Security Income—supplements Social Security payments based on need.

Veterans Health Administration
Website: *www.va.gov* (Click on Veteran Services, then Health Care.)
Phone: (800) 827-1000; healthcare benefits: (877) 222-8387

Eligible veterans and their dependents could receive cancer treatment and care at a Veterans Administration Medical Center.

Print publications
Landry, David S. *Be Prepared: The Complete Financial, Legal, and Practical Guide to Living with Cancer, HIV, and Other Life-Challenging Conditions.* New York: St. Martin's Press, 1998.

Financial Assistance Programs
Air Care Alliance
Website: *www.aircareall.org*
Phone: (888) 260-9707

Network of organizations willing to provide public benefit flights for health care.

Finding Ways to Pay for Care
(National Coalition for Cancer Survivorship)
Website: *www.canceradvocacy.org.*
(Select Cancer Resources and then Cancer Survival Toolbox.)

Partnership for Prescription Assistance
Website: *www.pparx.org*

Coalition of drug companies and other groups to help qualifying patients get the medicines they need for free or very low cost through public and private programs.

Hospice and End-of-Life Issues
Growth House
Website: *www.growthhouse.org*

Extensive annotated directory to hospice and end-of-life resources. Organized by topic.

Home Care Guide for Advanced Cancer
(American College of Physicians)
Website: *www.acponline.org*

Guide for family and friends caring for advanced cancer patients who are living at home.

Hospice Net
Website: *www.hospicenet.org*

Provides comprehensive information to patients and families facing life-threatening illness. Extensive resources addressing end-of-life issues from both patient and caregiver perspectives.

Patient Self-Advocacy Skills
Cancer Survival Toolbox
(National Coalition for Cancer Survivorship)
Website: *www.canceradvocacy.org* (Select Cancer Resources and then Cancer Survival Toolbox.)

Topics include communication skills, finding information, solving problems, making decisions, negotiating, and standing up for your rights. (Also available as audiotapes at (877) 866-5748.)

Questions to Ask Your Doctor
Website: *www.cancer.net* (Enter Doctor Questions in the search box.)

Physician and Hospital Locators
Finding the Best Lung Cancer Care
Website: *www.lungcanceronline.org*

Provides links to databases of lung cancer specialists (e.g., oncologists, thoracic surgeons) maintained by professional organizations and a listing of medical institutions that offer multidisciplinary lung cancer programs, including NCI-designated cancer centers.

Prevention and Risk Assessment

Cancer Research and Prevention Foundation

Website: *www.preventcancer.org*
Phone: (703) 836-4412; toll-free: (800) 227-2732
1600 Duke Street, Suite 500, Alexandria, VA 22314

Offers information on prevention and early detection of cancer.

Your Cancer Risk (Harvard School of Public Health)

Website: *www.diseaseriskindex.harvard.edu* (Click on Cancer.)

Online assessment tool that estimates your lung cancer risk and provides tips for prevention.

Research Resources and Reference

Dictionary of Cancer Terms (National Cancer Institute)

Website: *www.cancer.gov*

Medscape

Website: *www.medscape.com*. (Enter Lung Cancer in the search box.)

Medscape is an excellent source for the latest news in lung cancer research, including access to summaries of cancer conferences. Aimed at healthcare professionals. Registration required for free access to Medscape.

PubMed: MEDLINE (National Library of Medicine)

Website: *www.pubmed.org*

Provides free online access to MEDLINE, a database of more than 15 million citations to the medical literature.

Print Publications

Laughlin, EH. *Coming to Terms with Cancer: A Glossary of Cancer-Related Terms*. Atlanta, GA: American Cancer Society, 2002.

Smoking Cessation

Quitnet
Website: *www.quitnet.com*

Comprehensive Website for smoking cessation needs. Offers interactive personalized quitting tools, quitting guides, smoking cessation program locators, 24-hour online support/discussion, and links to smoking, tobacco, and cessation-related information and resources.

Smokefree.gov
Website: *www.smokefree.gov*

Information and professional assistance for people trying to quit smoking. Resources include cessation guides, telephone quit lines, instant messaging service, and print publications. Sponsored by the National Cancer Institute, the Centers for Disease Control, and the American Cancer Society.

Support Services

Association of Cancer Online Resources (ACOR)
Website: *www.acor.org* (Enter Lung Cancer in the search box.)

ACOR offers online support groups for cancer patients. Lung cancer lists include a general list (LUNG-ONC), lists for small cell lung cancer (LUNG-SCLC), lists for non-small cell lung cancer (LUNG-NSCLC), and lists for bronchioloalveolar (LUNG-BAC). Also offers a wide variety of support groups for general and specific cancer- and treatment-related issues.

CancerCare
Website: *www.cancercare.org*
Phone: (212) 712-8400; toll-free: (800) 813-4673
275 Seventh Avenue, New York, NY 10001

Provides comprehensive support services and programs to people with cancer.

National Lung Cancer Partnership
Website: *www.nationallungcancerpartnership.org*
Phone: (608) 233-7905
1 Point Place, Suite 200, Madison, WI 53719

Provides services under Living with Lung Cancer, such as educational materials, inspirational stories, blogs, and clinical trial information.

Phone Buddy Program (Lung Cancer Alliance)

Website:
www.lungcanceralliance.org (Enter Phone Buddy in the search box.)
Phone: (800) 298-2436

Offers peer-to-peer telephone support. Matches lung cancer survivors or their caregivers and family members with individuals who have faced, or are facing, similar circumstances.

R. A. Bloch National Cancer Foundation

Website: *www.blochcancer.org*
Phone: (816) 854-5050; toll-free: (800) 433-0464
4400 Main Street, Kansas City, MO 64111

Provides Bloch-authored cancer books free of charge, a multidisciplinary referral service, and patient-to-patient phone support.

Vital Options International

Website: *www.vitaloptions.org*
Phone: (818) 508-5657
4419 Coldwater Canyon Ave., Suite I, Studio City, CA 91604-1479

Produces "The Group Room," a weekly, syndicated radio call-in show (with simultaneous webcast) covering important and timely topics in cancer. Previous shows are archived for access on the Website.

Wellness Community

Website: *www.thewellnesscommunity.org*
Phone: (202) 659-9709; toll-free: (800) 793-WELL
1050 17th Street NW, Suite 500, Washington, DC 20036

Provides educational programs and support groups for people with cancer and their families.

Print Publications

Holland, JC and Lewis, S. *The Human Side of Cancer.* New York: Perennial Currents, 2001.

Schimmel, SR and Fox, B. *Cancer Talk: Voices of Hope and Endurance from "The Group Room," the World's Largest Cancer Support Group.* New York: Broadway Books, 1999.

St. John, Tina M. *With Every Breath: A Lung Cancer Guidebook.* The Lung Cancer Caring Ambassador's Program, 2005. Also available online at *www.lungcancerguidebook.org.*

Symptoms, Side Effects, and Complications

FATIGUE

CANCER-FATIGUE
(Association of Cancer Online Resources)
Website: *www.acor.org* (Enter Cancer Fatigue in the search box.)

Online discussion list covering cancer and treatment-related fatigue.

National Cancer Institute
Website: *www.cancer.gov* (Enter Fatigue in the search box.)
Phone: (800) 4-CANCER

American Cancer Society
Website: *www.cancer.org*
Phone: (800) ACS-2345

NCI/PDQ Fatigue
Website: *www.cancer.gov* (Enter Fatigue in the search box.)

Expert-reviewed information summary about cancer-related fatigue.

Print Publications
Harpham, WS. "Resolving the Frustration of Fatigue." *A Cancer Journal for Clinicians* 49(1999): 178–189.

Outstanding article by a patient/physician which discusses cancer-related fatigue and how to deal with it.

NAUSEA AND VOMITING

NCI/PDQ Nausea and Vomiting
Website: *www.cancer.gov* (Enter Nausea in the search box.)

Expert-reviewed information summary about nausea and vomiting related to cancer and its treatments.

NUTRITIONAL PROBLEMS

NCI/PDQ Nutrition
Website: *www.cancer.gov* (Enter Nutrition in the search box.)

Expert-reviewed information summary about the causes and management of nutritional problems occurring in cancer patients.

ORAL COMPLICATIONS

NCI/PDQ Oral Complications of Chemotherapy and Head/Neck Radiation
Website: *www.cancer.gov* (Enter Oral Complications in the search box.)

PAIN

NCI/PDQ Pain
Website: *www.cancer.gov* (Enter Pain in the search box.)

Expert-reviewed information summary about cancer-related pain. Includes discussion of approaches to the management and treatment of cancer-associated pain.

Print Publications
Abrahm, JL. *A Physician's Guide to Pain and Symptom Management in Cancer Patients*, Second Edition. Baltimore, MD: The Johns Hopkins University Press, 2005.

Aimed at healthcare professionals, this practical and comprehensive textbook is also an excellent resource for patients.

PERIPHERAL NEUROPATHY

The Neuropathy Association
Website: *www.neuropathy.org*
Phone: (212) 692-0662
60 East 42nd Street, Suite 942, New York, NY 10165

CANCER-NEUROPATHY
(Association of Cancer Online Resources)
Website: *www.acor.org* (Enter Cancer Neuropathy in the search box.)

Online discussion group for patients dealing with neuropathy induced by cancer or its treatments.

Print Publications
Almadrones, LA and R. Arcot. "Patient Guide to Peripheral Neuropathy." *Oncology Nursing Forum* 26, 8 (1999): 1359–1362.

PLEURAL EFFUSION

Sexual Effects
CANCER-FERTILITY and CANCER-SEXUALITY
(Association of Cancer Online Resources)
Website: *www.acor.org* (Enter Cancer Sexuality in the search box.)

Online discussion lists about fertility and sexuality issues associated with cancer.

NCI/PDQ Sexuality and Reproductive Issues
Website: *www.cancer.gov* (Enter Sexuality in the search box.)

Expert-reviewed information summary about factors that could affect fertility and sexual functioning in people who have cancer.

Tests and Procedures
Cancer Imaging (National Cancer Institute)
Website: *www.cancer.gov* (Enter Cancer Imaging in the search box.)

Laboratory Tests (MEDLINEplus)
Website: *www.nlm.nih.gov*

Print Publications

Margolis, S., ed. *The Johns Hopkins Consumer Guide to Medical Tests: What You Can Expect, How You Should Prepare, What Your Results Mean.* New York City, NU: Rebus, Inc., 2001.

Treatment Information and Guidelines

NCI/PDQ Non-small Cell Lung Cancer Treatment and Small Cell Lung Cancer Treatment

Website: *www.cancer.gov* (Enter Lung Cancer in the search box and then select the first suggested link.)

Expert-reviewed summaries about the treatment of NSCLC and SCLC.

Chemotherapy and You (NIH/NCI)

Website: *www.cancer.gov* (Enter Chemotherapy and You in the search box.) Also available in print by calling (800) 4CANCER.

Radiation Therapy and You (NIH/NCI)

Website: *www.cancer.gov* (Enter Radiation Therapy and You in the search box.) Also available in print by calling (800) 4CANCER.

Surgery for Lung Cancer (CancerHelp UK)

Website: *www.cancerhelp.org.uk* (Enter Surgery for Lung Cancer in the search box.)

Survivorship Issues

LT-SURVIVORS (Association of Cancer Online Resources)

Website: *www.acor.org* (Enter Long-term Survivors in the serach box.) Forum for discussion of issues of concern to long-term cancer survivors.

National Coalition for Cancer Survivorship (NCCS)

Website: *www.canceradvocacy.org*
Phone: (301) 650-9127; toll-free: (877) NCCS-YES
1010 Wayne Avenue, Suite 770, Silver Spring, MD 20910

Print Publications

Harpham, WS. *After Cancer: A Guide to Your New Life*. New York: Perennial Currents, 1995.

Women and People of Color

National Lung Cancer Partnership
Website: *www.nationallungcancerpartnership.org*
Phone: (608) 233-7905
1 Point Place, Suite 200, Madison, WI 53719

Office of Minority Health
Website: *www.minorityhealth.hhs.gov*
Phone: (240) 453-2882
1101 Wootton Parkway, Suite 600, Rockville, MD 20852

WomensHealth.gov
Website: *www.womenshealth.gov*
Phone: (202) 690-7650
200 Independence Avenue, SW, Washington, DC 20201

A

Adenocarcinoma: A type of non-small cell lung cancer; a malignant tumor that arises from glandular tissue.

Adenocarcinoma-in-situ (AIS): Formerly called bronchoalveolar carcinoma, a subtype of adenocarcinoma sometimes found in non-smokers.

Adjuvant chemotherapy: Therapy given after surgery in case any cancer cells have been left behind.

Advance directives: Legal documents that allow you to prepare for future medical possibilities and to assign someone to act on your behalf in the event you become unable to direct your own medical care.

Alopecia: Hair loss.

Alveoli: Tiny air sacs that compose the lungs.

Anemia: Low red blood cell count; may cause tiredness, weakness, and shortness of breath.

Angiogenesis: The formation of new blood vessels that allows tumors to grow.

Angiogenesis inhibitors: Drugs that prevent the formation of new blood vessels.

Antiemetics: Drugs that prevent nausea and vomiting.

Apoptosis: Process by which normal cells die when they are injured; often referred to as programmed cell death.

Arm of a clinical study: Treatment group to which a patient is assigned in a randomized clinical trial.

Asymptomatic: Without symptoms.

B

Benign: Not cancerous; not life threatening.

Biopsy: Removal of tissue or fluid sample for microscopic examination.

Biostatistician: A statistician who specialize in the study of the natural variations found in biology and the natural world.

Bone scan: An imaging test in which a radionuclear substance is injected into the veins and taken up by the bones in areas of potential metastatic disease.

Brachytherapy: Internal radiation therapy that involves placing seeds of radioactive material near or in the tumor.

Bronchioloalveolar carcinoma (now called **Adenocarcinoma-in-situ [AIS]**): A type of adenocarcinoma.

Bronchoscope: See **Bronchoscopy**.

Bronchoscopy: A procedure that involves inserting a flexible tube (**bronchoscope**) through the nose down into the lungs. Needles can be inserted through the bronchoscope to obtain biopsy samples.

C

Carcinogenesis: The development of cancer.

Carcinogens: Cancer-causing substances.

Cells: Microscopic units that make up the organs of the body.

Centigray: Unit of radiation; same as a rad.

Central venous catheter (CVC): A thin tube that is surgically inserted to allow access to large veins.

Chemoprevention: The use of natural or synthetic substances to prevent cancer.

Chemopreventive agent: A natural or synthetic substance used to prevent cancer.

Chemotherapy: The use of medicine to treat cancer; a whole-body or systemic treatment.

Chromosomes: Strands of DNA and proteins in the cell nucleus that are composed of a series of genes.

Chronic obstructive pulmonary disease (COPD): Chronic bronchitis or emphysema.

Clinical trials: Research studies involving people.

Clubbing: A condition that causes the nails on the fingers to bulge out; clubbing occurs with many different types of lung problems.

Colony-stimulating factors: Substances that stimulate bone marrow to increase production of blood cells; also referred to as growth factors.

Complementary and alternative medicine (CAM): Therapies developed outside of mainstream medicine and used in place of standard, clinically proven therapies.

Complete blood count (CBC): A blood test that counts the number of white blood cells, red blood cells, and platelets.

Complete response: The disappearance of all signs of cancer in response to treatment. This does not always mean the cancer has been cured. Also called complete remission.

COPD: Chronic obstructive pulmonary disease. Emphysema and bronchitis are the two most common forms of COPD.

CT scan (computed tomography): Computerized series of X-rays that create a detailed cross-sectional image of the body.

Cranial irradiation: The exposure of the head to roentgen rays or other forms of radioactivity for therapeutic or preventive purposes.

Curative treatment: Treatment given with the intent to cure the patient of his or her cancer.

Cycle: The schedule of administration of chemotherapy that is repeated four–six times.

D

Deep vein thrombosis (DVT): A blood clot occurring in a deep-lying vein in the leg or pelvis.

Differentiation: A term used to describe the degree to which tumor tissue resembles normal tissue.

DNA (deoxyribonucleic acid): Molecules that make up genes.

Do Not Resuscitate (DNR) order: An advance directive stating you do not want doctors to do whatever is necessary to keep you alive in the event of a cardiac or respiratory arrest.

Doublet chemotherapy: Two chemotherapy drugs used together.

Driver mutation: A mutation which causes a cancer cell to grow and divide; without this specific mutation, the cancer cell would die.

Durable power of attorney for health care: An advance directive that allows you to specify a healthcare proxy to make medical decisions for you should you become unable to do so for yourself.

E

Electrolytes: Acids, bases, and salts essential for maintaining life; electrolyte abnormalities are imbalances of salts or chemicals in the blood.

EGFR: The receptor on the surface of the cancer cell to which EGF binds.

EML-4/ALK fusion protein: An abnormal protein made when two genes combine (e.g., the EML-4 gene and the ALK gene). The resulting protein can cause cancer cells to grow and divide.

Epidermal growth factor (EGF): A protein made by cancer cells that causes cancer cells around them to grow and divide.

Esophagus: The tube through which food travels from the mouth to the stomach.

External CVCs: IVs inserted in a large blood vessel. The other end is exposed through the skin and capped off so a patient does not have to carry an IV bag with them all the time.

F

Fibrosis: Scarring.

First-line therapy: Initial treatment.

Fraction: Single treatment of radiation. The total dose of radiation is usually given over multiple fractions.

G

Gene: A section or sequence of DNA that regulates specific functions and is located in a specific place on a chromosome.

Genomics: The study of all mutations in a tumor to identify patterns that can be used to predict which tumors are more or less likely to respond to chemotherapy.

Gray (Gy): Modern unit of radiation dosage. 100 rads is equal to one Gy.

Growth factors: Substances that stimulate cells to grow; drugs that help the bone marrow recover from the effects of chemotherapy (see also colony-stimulating factors).

Growth factor inhibitors: Substances that inhibit the growth factors that stimulate cells to grow.

H

Healthcare proxy: A person you have designated to make healthcare decisions for you in the event you become incapacitated.

Hematocrit: The proportion of the blood that consists of red blood cells.

Hemoglobin: The oxygen-carrying protein in the red blood cells.

Hemoptysis: Coughing up blood.

Hilar lymph nodes: Lymph nodes located in the region where the bronchus meets the lung.

Histological: Tissue type; assessment of cellular features by microscopic evaluation.

Hospice: An organization that provides end-of-life care that focuses on palliative rather than curative care and provides a wide range of support to dying patients and their families.

I

Incidence: The number of new cases of a cancer (or any disease or event) in a defined population during a set period of time.

Informed consent: A process that provides potential participants in a clinical trial the information they need to make an informed decision about whether or not to participate.

Intensity Modulated Radiation Therapy (IMRT): A type of three-dimensional radiation therapy (3D-CRT) that uses radiation beams of varying strengths.

Interventional radiologist: A radiologist who uses X-rays and other imaging techniques to perform minimally invasive medical procedures.

Intravenous: In the vein.

L

Large cell carcinoma: A type of non-small cell lung cancer.

Ligand: A molecule that binds to another chemical entity to form a larger complex.

Linac: A linear accelerator that produces high-energy X-rays for radiation therapy.

Living will: A document in which you specify which medical treatments you do and do not want to have should you become unable to decide for yourself.

Lobectomy: Surgical removal of a lobe of the lung.

Lobes: Clear anatomical divisions or extensions that can be determined without the use of a microscope (at the gross anatomy level). The right lung contains three lobes and the left contains two.

Lymph node: Small collections of white blood cells scattered throughout the body.

Lymph node dissection: Surgical removal of lymph nodes.

Lymphatic system: A vascular system that contains lymph nodes through which white blood cells flow; cancer can also spread through the lymphatic system.

M

Main stem bronchi: The two main breathing tubes (right main stem bronchus and left main stem bronchus) that branch off the trachea.

Maintenance therapy: A single drug given indefinitely after standard doublet chemotherapy to maintain the remission.

Malignant: Cancerous; cells that exhibit rapid, uncontrolled growth and can spread to other parts of the body.

Mediastinal lymph nodes: Lymph nodes located in the mediastinum, the area between the lungs.

Mediastinoscopy: A surgical procedure by which lymph nodes can be removed for microscopic examination.

Mediastinum: Area between the lungs.

Medical oncologist: A physician who performs comprehensive management of cancer patients throughout all phases of care; specializes in treating cancer with medicine.

Metastasis: The spread of cancer from the initial cancer site to other parts of the body.

Minimally invasive surgery: Surgery which uses smaller incisions than a regular operation and thus is less painful for the patient post-operatively. In order to be able to operate through such a small incision, the surgeon must used advanced, fibro electronic instruments.

Mortality: The number of people who die of a disease.

Multidisciplinary clinic: One in which doctors of different specialities—e.g., medical oncology, radiation oncology and surgeons—all see the patient within the same clinic.

Mutation: A damaged gene.

Myelosuppression: A decrease in the production of blood cells.

N

N1 nodes: Hilar nodes (e.g., nodes at the base of the lung).

N2 nodes: Mediastinal nodes (e.g., nodes between the lungs and the heart).

Nadir: Lowest measured value; period of low blood counts.

Negative margins: A phrase used when normal tissue is found at the edge of the biopsy sample.

Neoadjuvant chemotherapy: Therapy given before the primary therapy; for example, neoadjuvant chemotherapy, which is sometimes given prior to surgery.

Neuropathy: See **peripheral neuropathy**.

Neutropenia: Low white blood cell count.

Neutrophil: A type of white blood cell that attacks bacteria.

Nicotine replacement therapy: Smoking cessation method that uses nicotine substitutes in various forms, including a patch, gum, inhaler, or nasal spray.

Non-small cell lung cancer (NSCLC): A type of lung cancer that includes adenocarcinoma, squamous cell carcinoma, and large cell carcinoma.

Nucleus: The center of the cell.

Nutritionist or dietician: A person trained to provide nutritional or dietary counseling.

O

Oncogene: A gene that, when mutated, can allow a cell to grow uncontrollably.

Oncology nurse: A specialized nurse trained to provide care to cancer patients.

Oncology social worker: A social worker trained to provide counseling and practical assistance to cancer patients.

P

Palliation: Reducing symptoms.

Palliative care specialist: A physician trained in management of pain or other symptoms of cancer.

Palliative treatment: Treatment given not with the intent to cure but with the intent to prolong survival and reduce symptoms from the tumor.

Pancoast tumor (superior sulcus tumor): A tumor occurring near the top of the lungs that may cause shoulder pain or weakness or a group of symptoms including a droopy eyelid, dry eyes, and lack of sweating on the face.

Paraneoplastic symptoms: Symptoms that result from substances released by cancer cells and that occur at a site not directly involved with the tumor.

Parietal pleura: A membrane lining the chest wall.

Partial response: A decrease in the size of a tumor, or in the extent of cancer in the body, in response to treatment. Also called **partial remission**.

Passive smoking: Inhaling cigarette smoke of others.

Pathologist: A physician trained to examine and evaluate cells and tissue.

Patient-controlled analgesia (PCA): A method by which a patient can regulate the amount of pain medication he or she receives.

Patient navigator: A nurse, nurse practitioner, social worker, or other healthcare personnel whose job is to coordinate your care (e.g., make sure all your questions are answered, your tests are scheduled, your treatments are on time, etc.)

Performance status: The general condition and activity level of the patient.

Pericardial effusion: Accumulation of fluid inside the sac (pericardium) that surrounds the heart.

Pericardium: A double-layered serous membrane that surrounds the heart.

Peripheral neuropathy: Tingling, numbness, or burning sensation in hands, feet, or legs caused by damage to peripheral nerves by a tumor or by chemotherapy or radiation.

Personalized medicine: Treatment of a patient not based upon where it arose, but upon the molecular characterization of the tumor, so that each patient will get a treatment designed specifically for them based upon the molecular characteristics of the tumor.

PET scan (positron emission tomography): A nuclear medicine imaging test that measures metabolism; often used to differentiate between healthy and abnormal (e.g., cancerous) tissue.

Phlebotomist: A technician trained to draw blood.

Pic-line: a type of central venous catheter inserted into a large vein in the arm.

Placebo: An inactive substance (e.g., sugar pill). Placebos alone are rarely used in cancer trials.

Platelet: A type of blood cell responsible for clotting.

Platin doublet: One of the two drugs in the doublet is either cisplatin or carboplatin.

Pleural effusion: Accumulation of fluid between the outside of the lung and the inside of the chest wall.

Pleural space: The area between the outside of the lung and the inside of the chest wall.

Pleurex catheter: Provides symptomatic relief of dyspnea related to recurrent pleural effusions.

Pleurodesis: A procedure to prevent recurrence of pleural effusion by draining the fluid and inserting medication into the pleural space.

Pneumonectomy: Surgical removal of the entire lung.

Pneumonia: An infection of the lung.

Pneumonitis: Irritation of the lungs.

Poorly differentiated: Cancer cells that look wildly abnormal and nothing like the organ they started in.

Port: A type of central venous catheter that is surgically implanted under the skin.

Positive margins: A phrase used when cancer cells are found at the edge of the biopsy sample.

Prognosis: Predicted outcome; likelihood of survival.

Prophylactic cranial irradiation (PCI): Radiation to the brain with the intention of preventing the development of brain metastases.

Psychiatrist: A physician who specializes in treating people for depression, anxiety, and other psychological illness. Psychiatrists provide psychotherapy and can also prescribe medication.

Psychologist: A person trained in psychology who can provide psychotherapy or counseling to help patients and their families better cope with their disease.

Pulmonary embolism (PE): A blood clot that travels to the lungs causing full or partial blockage of one or both pulmonary arteries.

Pulmonary function tests (PFTs): A group of breathing tests used to determine lung health.

Pulmonologist: A physician who specializes in the diagnosis and treatment of lung diseases.

R

Rad: Unit of radiation.

Radiation fibrosis: Scarring of the lungs caused by radiation treatment.

Radiation oncologist: A physician who specializes in treating cancer with radiation.

Radiation therapy: Treatment that uses high-dose X-rays or other high-energy rays to kill cancer cells.

Radiofrequency ablation (RFA): Treatment that uses high-frequency electric current to kill cancer cells.

Radioprotectant: A medication that reduces certain side effects of radiation.

Radiotherapy: The treatment of disease with ionizing radiation. Also called **radiation therapy.**

Randomized controlled trial (RCT): A research study in which the participants are assigned by chance (using a computer) to separate groups that compare different treatments; a method used to prevent bias in research.

Receptor: A protein molecule, embedded in either the plasma membrane or cytoplasm of a cell, to which a signaling molecule (or ligand) may attach.

Red blood cell (RBC): The most common type of blood cell and the body's principal means of delivering oxygen to the body tissues via the blood.

Regimen: Specific chemotherapy treatment plan involving the drugs, doses, and frequency of administration.

Rehabilitation specialist: A person trained to help patients recover from physical changes brought about by cancer or cancer treatment.

Remission: Shrinkage of tumor in response to treatment. May be either complete (total disappearance of tumor) or partial (the tumor has shrunk, but has not gone away entirely).

Resectable: Able to be surgically removed (resected).

Resection: Surgical removal.

Respiratory depression: Slowing of breathing.

Responding: Cancer that has shrunk in response to chemotherapy.

Robotic surgery: A type of minimally invasive surgery, in which the surgeon manipulates the instruments from a console that does not have to be next to the patient's bed.

S

Schedule: How frequently chemotherapy is given.

Second-line treatment: Treatment method(s) used following an initial treatment that either does not stop cancer progression or stops it only temporarily.

Signatures: Patterns of expression of many genes or proteins, which is unique to that type of cancer.

Simulation: Planning the radiation fields with a CT scan.

Small cell carcinoma: A type of lung cancer that differs in appearance and behavior from non-small cell lung cancers (adenocarcinoma, squamous cell carcinoma, large cell carcinoma).

Small cell lung cancer (SCLC): Refers to small cell carcinoma, as opposed to non-small cell lung cancers (adenocarcinoma, squamous cell carcinoma, large cell carcinoma).

Sputum: Mucus and other secretions produced by the lungs.

Squamous cell carcinoma: A type of non-small cell lung cancer.

Stable: Cancer has stopped growing following treatment.

Staging: Determining the size of a cancer and how far it has spread.

Stent: A hollow tube that can be inserted via bronchoscopy into the airway to prevent it from being blocked or crushed by the tumor.

Stereotactic Body Radiation Therapy (SBRT): A way of delivering very high doses of radiation to the tumor in 3–5 fractions, without damaging surrounding normal tissues.

Superior sulcus tumor: See **pancoast tumor**.

Superior vena cava syndrome (SVCS): A collection of symptoms that could include swelling in the neck, shoulders, and arms caused by a lung tumor pressing on the SVC, one of the large vessels leading into the heart.

Surgery: Removal of tissue by means of an operation (surgical procedure).

Systemic: Affecting the entire body.

T

T4: A tumor that invades the mediastinum, heart, ribs or spine, or any of the major structures in the chest OR has spread to another area in the same lobe.

Targetable mutation: A mutation against which a drug can be made.

Targeted therapy: Therapy directed at aspects of the cell that are specific for cancer.

Thoracentesis: A procedure that uses a needle to remove fluid from the space between the lung and the chest wall.

Thoracic surgeon: A surgeon who specializes in performing chest surgery.

Thoracotomy: A common type of lung surgery that requires a large incision to provide access to the lungs.

Three-dimensional conformal radiation therapy (3D-CRT): A type of radiation therapy that enables higher doses of radiation to be delivered more precisely than standard radiation therapy.

Thrombocytopenia: Low counts of platelets that could result in bruising and/or bleeding.

Trachea: Breathing tube (airway) leading from the larynx to the lungs.

Transthoracic (percutaneous) biopsy: A biopsy obtained by inserting a needle through the skin and chest wall into the tumor.

Treatment field: The area of the body that is radiated.

TTF1: A protein lung adenocarcinoma cells have on the outside of their membrane. Since it is primarily found on adenocarcinoma cells of the lung, and not other types of cancer, it is frequently used to tell if a cancer in the lung started in the lung (e,g., lung cancer) or whether it spread to the lung from some other organ (e.g., metastatsized to the lung).

Tumor: A mass of tissue formed by a new growth of cells.

Tumor suppressor gene: A gene that can normally block cancer from developing; when mutated, it cannot stop the growth of abnormal cells.

Tyrosine kinase inhibitors (TKIs): Small molecules which block the activated part of the receptor on the inside of the cancer cell and prevent it from starting a chemical reaction which causes the cell to grow and divide.

V

VEGF (vascular endothelial growth factor): A family of growth factors, most often made by tumors, that causes blood vessel cells (vascular cells) to grow into the tumor.

Video-assisted thoracoscopic surgery (VATS): A type of minimally invasive chest surgery.

Visceral pleura: A membrane surrounding the lung.

X

X-ray: High-energy radiation used to image the body.

W

Wedge resection: Surgical removal of the tumor and a small amount of lung tissue surrounding the tumor.

Well-differentiated: Cancer cells which look relatively similar to the organ in which they started.

White blood cells: A type of blood cell that fights infection.